Essential Psych

The Pres
Gu

D0924506

ANTIPSYCHOTICS AND MOOD STABILIZERS

New!

In response to the rapid developments in psychopharmacology, this is a spin-off from Stephen Stahl's new, completely revised and updated edition of his much acclaimed *Prescriber's Guide.* It covers the most important drugs in use today for psychosis and mood stabilization.

In full color throughout, and with four or more pages for each of the antipsychotic drugs, Stephen Stahl distills his great expertise into a pragmatic formulary that gives all the information a prescriber needs to treat patients effectively. Each drug is covered in five categories: • *general therapeutics,* • *dosing and use,* • *side effects,* • *special populations,* and • *pearls.*

Target icons appear next to key categories for each drug so that the prescriber can go easily and instantly to the information needed. Two indexes are included, listing drugs by name (generic and international) and use. In addition Dr. Stahl indicates which drugs have FDA approval, and also gives the FDA Use-in-Pregnancy Ratings.

Stephen M. Stahl is Adjunct Professor of Psychiatry at the University of California, San Diego. He has conducted numerous research projects awarded by the National Institute of Mental Health, the Veteran's Administration, and the pharmaceutical industry. The author of more than 300 articles and chapters, Stephen Stahl is an internationally recognized clinician, researcher, and teacher in psychiatry with subspecialty expertise in psychopharmacology.

From reviews of the first *Prescriber's Guide:*

". . . instead of a laundry list, Dr. Stahl presents what the clinician ought to be looking for – this is not your father's PDR (*Physician's Desk Reference*)! The clinical tips and pearls that are found in each entry are invaluable – not only are dosing guidelines provided, but also the author's educated and respected opinion regarding potential advantages and disadvantages of each drug . . . a real bargain. . . . The book's major strength is its readability and user friendliness. The art of psychopharmacology is finally given the space it deserves. . . . This guidebook is an excellent source of information for the art of prescribing psychotropic medications and belongs in every clinician's library."
The Annals of Pharmacotherapy

"I think that this manual has all the characteristics of a true bestseller. The format is very attractive, the information is complete, the consultation is easy. In no other recent text will a clinician find so much information in such a concise and user-friendly format."
Acta Psychiatrica Scandinavica, reviewer Mario Maj

Essential Psychopharmacology

The Prescriber's Guide

ANTIPSYCHOTICS AND MOOD STABILIZERS

Stephen M. Stahl, M.D., Ph.D.

Adjunct Professor of Psychiatry
University of California at San Diego

Editorial assistant
Meghan M. Grady

With illustrations by
Nancy Muntner

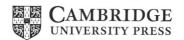

CAMBRIDGE
UNIVERSITY PRESS

Every effort has been made in preparing this book to provide accurate and up-to-date information that is in accord with accepted standards and practice at the time of publication. Nevertheless, the author, editors and publisher can make no warranties that the information contained herein is totally free from error, not least because clinical standards are constantly changing through research and regulation. The authors, editors and publisher therefore disclaim all liability for direct or consequential damages resulting from the use of material contained in this book. Readers are strongly advised to pay careful attention to information provided by the manufacturer of any drugs or equipment that they plan to use.

PUBLISHED BY CAMBRIDGE UNIVERSITY PRESS
Cambridge, New York, Melbourne, Madrid, Cape Town, Singapore, São Paulo

CAMBRIDGE UNIVERSITY PRESS
20 West 20th Street, New York NY, 10011-4211 USA
www.cambridge.org

Information on this title: www.cambridge.org/9780521616355

First published 2006

Printed in Canada by Friesens

*A catalog record for this book is available from
the British Library*

Library of Congress Cataloging-in-Publication Data

Stahl, S. M.
    Essential psychopharmacology : the prescriber's guide. Antipsychotics and
mood stabilizers / Stephen M. Stahl ; editorial assistant, Meghan M. Grady
; with illustrations by Nancy Muntner.
        p. ; cm.
    Includes index.
    ISBN-13: 978-0-521-61635-5 (pbk.)
    ISBN-10: 0-521-61635-2 (pbk.)
    1. Antipsychotic drugs--Handbooks, manuals, etc. 2. Affective
disorders--Chemotherapy--Handbooks, manuals, etc. 3.
Psychoses--Chemotherapy--Handbooks, manuals, etc.
    [DNLM: 1. Antipsychotic Agents--therapeutic use--Handbooks. 2. Mood
Disorders--drug therapy--Handbooks. 3. Psychotic Disorders--drug
therapy--Handbooks. QV 39 S781ec 2006] I. Title: Antipsychotics and mood
stabilizers. II. Title.

    RM333.5.S736 2006
    615'.7882--dc22

To members of the Neuroscience Education Institute and prescribers of psychopharmacologic agents everywhere. Your relentless determination to find the best portfolio of treatments for each individual patient within your practice is my inspiration.

Table of contents

Introduction

This *Guide* is intended to complement *Essential Psychopharmacology*. *Essential Psychopharmacology* emphasizes mechanisms of action and how psychotropic drugs work upon receptors and enzymes in the brain. This *Guide* gives practical information on how to use antipsychotics and mood stabilizers in clinical practice.

It would be impossible to include all available information about any drug in a single work and no attempt is made here to be comprehensive. The purpose of this *Guide* is instead to integrate the art of clinical practice with the science of psychopharmacology. That means including only essential facts in order to keep things short. Unfortunately that also means excluding less critical facts as well as extraneous information, which may nevertheless be useful to the reader but would make the book too long and dilute the most important information. In deciding what to include and what to omit, the author has drawn upon common sense and 30 years of clinical experience with patients. He has also consulted with many experienced clinicians and analysed the evidence from controlled clinical trials and regulatory filings with government agencies.

In order to meet the needs of the clinician and to facilitate future updates of this *Guide*, the opinions of readers are sincerely solicited. Feedback can be emailed to feedback@neiglobal.com. Specifically, are the best and most essential antipsychotics and mood stabilizers included here? Do you find any factual errors? Are there agreements or disagreements with any of the opinions expressed here? Are there suggestions for any additional tips or pearls for future editions? Any and all suggestions and comments are welcomed.

All of the selected drugs are presented in the same design format in order to facilitate rapid access to information. Specifically, each drug is broken down into five sections, each designated by a unique color background: ■ therapeutics, ■ side effects, ■ dosing and use, ■ special populations, and ■ the art of psychopharmacology, followed by key references.

Therapeutics covers the brand names in major countries; the class of drug; what it is commonly prescribed and approved for by the United States Food and Drug Administration (FDA); how the drug works; how long it takes to work; what to do if it works or if it doesn't work; the best augmenting combinations for partial response or treatment resistance, and the tests (if any) that are required.

Side effects explains how the drug causes side effects; gives a list of notable, life threatening or dangerous side effects; gives a specific rating for weight gain or sedation, and advice about how to handle side effects, including best augmenting agents for side effects.

Dosing and use gives the usual dosing range; dosage forms; how to dose and dosing tips; symptoms of overdose; long-term use; if habit forming, how to stop; pharmacokinetics; drug interactions; when not to use and other warnings or precautions.

Special populations gives specific information about any possible renal, hepatic and cardiac impairments, and any precautions to be taken for treating the elderly, children, adolescents, and pregnant and breast-feeding women.

The art of psychopharmacology gives the author's opinions on issues such as the potential advantages and disadvantages of any one drug, the primary target symptoms, and clinical pearls to get the best out of a drug.

At the back of the *Guide* are two indexes. The first is an index by drug name, giving both generic names (uncapitalized) and trade names (capitalized and followed by the generic name in parentheses). The second is an index of common uses for the generic drugs included in the *Guide* and is organized by disorder/symptom. Agents that are approved by the FDA for a particular use are shown in bold. In addition to these indexes there is a list of abbreviations; FDA definitions for the Pregnancy Categories A, B, C, D and X, and, finally, an index of the icons used in the *Guide*.

Readers are encouraged to consult standard references[1] and comprehensive psychiatry and pharmacology textbooks for more in-depth information. They are also reminded that the art of psychopharmacology section is the author's opinion.

It is strongly advised that readers familiarize themselves with the standard use of these drugs before attempting any of the more exotic uses discussed, such as unusual drug combinations and doses. Reading about both drugs before augmenting one with the other is also strongly recommended. Today's psychopharmacologist should also regularly track blood pressure, weight and body mass index for most of their patients. The dutiful clinician will also check out the drug interactions of non-central-nervous-system (CNS) drugs with those that act in the CNS, including any prescribed by other clinicians.

Certain drugs, such as clozapine, may be for experts only. Off-label uses not approved by the FDA and inadequately studied doses or combinations of drugs may also be for the expert only, who can weigh risks and benefits in the presence of sometimes vague and conflicting evidence. Pregnant or nursing women, or people with two or more psychiatric illnesses, substance abuse, and/or a concomitant medical illness may be suitable patients for the expert only. Use your best judgement as to your level of expertise and realize that we are all learning in this rapidly advancing field. The practice of medicine is often not so much a science as it is an art. It is important to stay within the standards of medical care for the field, and also within your personal comfort zone, while trying to help extremely ill and often difficult patients with medicines that can sometimes transform their lives and relieve their suffering.

Finally, this book is intended to be genuinely helpful for practitioners of psychopharmacology by providing them with the mixture of facts and opinions selected by the author. Ultimately, prescribing choices are the reader's responsibility. Every effort has been made in preparing this book to provide accurate and up-to-date information in accord with accepted standards and practice at the time of publication. Nevertheless, the psychopharmacology field is evolving rapidly and the author and publisher make no warranties that the information contained herein is totally free from error, not least because clinical standards are constantly changing through research and regulation. Furthermore, the author and publisher disclaim any responsibility for the continued currency of this information and disclaim all liability for any and all damages, including direct or consequential damages, resulting from the use of information contained in this book. Doctors recommending and patients using these drugs are strongly advised to pay careful attention to, and consult information provided by the manufacturer.

---

[1] For example, *Physician's Desk Reference* and *Martindale's*

List of icons

 alpha 2 agonist

 anticonvulsant

 antihistamine

 benzodiazepine

 cholinesterase inhibitor

 conventional antipsychotic

 dopamine stabilizer

 lithium

 modafinil (wake-promoter)

 monoamine oxidase inhibitor

 nefazodone (serotonin antagonist/reuptake inhibitor)

 N-methyl-d-aspartate antagonist

 noradrenergic and specific serotonergic antidepressant

norepinephrine and dopamine reuptake inhibitor

 sedative hypnotic

 selective norepinephrine reuptake inhibitor

 selective serotonin reuptake inhibitor

 serotonin-dopamine antagonist

 serotonin and norepinephrine reuptake inhibitor

 serotonin 1A partial agonist

 stimulant

 trazodone (serotonin antagonist/reuptake inhibitor)

 tricyclic/tetracyclic antidepressant

 How the drug works, mechanism of action

 Best augmenting agents to add for partial response or treatment-resistance

 Life-threatening or dangerous side effects

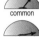

Weight Gain: Degrees of weight gain associated with the drug, with unusual signifying that weight gain has been reported but is not expected; not unusual signifying that weight gain occurs in a significant minority; common signifying that many experience weight gain and/or it can be significant in amount; and problematic signifying that weight gain occurs frequently, can be significant in amount, and may be a health problem in some patients

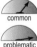

Sedation: Degrees of sedation associated with the drug, with unusual signifying that sedation has been reported but is not expected; not unusual signifying that sedation occurs in a significant minority; common signifying that many experience sedation and/or it can be significant in amount; and problematic signifying that sedation occurs frequently, can be significant in amount, and may be a health problem in some patients

Tips for dosing based on the clinical expertise of the author

Drug interactions that may occur

Warnings and precautions regarding use of the drug

Dosing and other information specific to children and adolescents

Information regarding use of the drug during pregnancy

Clinical pearls of information based on the clinical expertise of the author

AMISULPRIDE

THERAPEUTICS

Brands • Solian
see index for additional brand names

Generic? No

Class
• Atypical antipsychotic (benzamide; possibly a dopamine stabilizer and dopamine partial agonist)

Commonly Prescribed For
(bold for FDA approved)
• Schizophrenia, acute and chronic (outside of U.S., especially Europe)
• Dysthymia

How The Drug Works
• Theoretically blocks presynaptic dopamine 2 receptors at low doses
• Theoretically blocks postsynaptic dopamine 2 receptors at higher doses
* May be a partial agonist at dopamine 2 receptors, which would theoretically reduce dopamine output when dopamine concentrations are high and increase dopamine output when dopamine concentrations are low
• Blocks dopamine 3 receptors, which may contribute to its clinical actions
* Unlike other atypical antipsychotics, amisulpride does not have potent actions at serotonin receptors

How Long Until It Works
• Psychotic symptoms can improve within 1 week, but it may take several weeks for full effect on behavior as well as on cognition and affective stabilization
• Classically recommended to wait at least 4–6 weeks to determine efficacy of drug, but in practice some patients require up to 16–20 weeks to show a good response, especially on cognitive symptoms

If It Works
• Most often reduces positive symptoms in schizophrenia but does not eliminate them
• Can improve negative symptoms, as well as aggressive, cognitive, and affective symptoms in schizophrenia
• Most schizophrenic patients do not have a total remission of symptoms but rather a reduction of symptoms by about a third
• Perhaps 5–15% of schizophrenic patients can experience an overall improvement of greater than 50–60%, especially when receiving stable treatment for more than a year
• Such patients are considered super-responders or "awakeners" since they may be well enough to be employed, live independently, and sustain long-term relationships
• Continue treatment until reaching a plateau of improvement
• After reaching a satisfactory plateau, continue treatment for at least a year after first episode of psychosis
• For second and subsequent episodes of psychosis, treatment may need to be indefinite
• Even for first episodes of psychosis, it may be preferable to continue treatment indefinitely to avoid subsequent episodes

If It Doesn't Work
• Try one of the other first-line atypical antipsychotics (risperidone, olanzapine, quetiapine, ziprasidone, aripiprazole)
• If two or more antipsychotic monotherapies do not work, consider clozapine
• If no atypical antipsychotic is effective, consider higher doses or augmentation with valproate or lamotrigine
• Some patients may require treatment with a conventional antipsychotic
• Consider noncompliance and switch to another antipsychotic with fewer side effects or to an antipsychotic that can be given by depot injection
• Consider initiating rehabilitation and psychotherapy
• Consider presence of concomitant drug abuse

Best Augmenting Combos for Partial Response or Treatment-Resistance
• Valproic acid (valproate, divalproex, divalproex ER)
• Augmentation of amisulpride has not been systematically studied

- Other mood stabilizing anticonvulsants (carbamazepine, oxcarbazepine, lamotrigine)
- Lithium
- Benzodiazepines

Tests

❋ Although risk of diabetes and dyslipidemia with amisulpride has not been systematically studied, monitoring as for all other atypical antipsychotics is suggested

Before starting an atypical antipsychotic

❋ Weigh all patients and track BMI during treatment
- Get baseline personal and family history of diabetes, obesity, dyslipidemia, hypertension, and cardiovascular disease
- Get waistline circumference (at umbilicus), blood pressure, fasting plasma glucose, and fasting lipid profile
- Determine if patient is
  - overweight (BMI 25.0–29.9)
  - obese (BMI ≥30)
  - has pre-diabetes (fasting plasma glucose 100–125 mg/dl)
  - has diabetes (fasting plasma glucose >126 mg/dl)
  - has hypertension (BP >140/90 mm Hg)
  - has dyslipidemia (increased total cholesterol, LDL cholesterol, and triglycerides; decreased HDL cholesterol)
- Treat or refer such patients for treatment, including nutrition and weight management, physical activity counseling, smoking cessation, and medical management

Monitoring after starting an atypical antipsychotic

❋ BMI monthly for 3 months, then quarterly
- Blood pressure, fasting plasma glucose, fasting lipids within 3 months and then annually, but earlier and more frequently for patients with diabetes or who have gained >5% initial weight
- Treat or refer for treatment and consider switching to another atypical antipsychotic for patients who become overweight, obese, pre-diabetic, diabetic, hypertensive, or dyslipidemic while receiving an atypical antipsychotic
❋ Even in patients without known diabetes, be vigilant for the rare but life threatening onset of diabetic ketoacidosis, which always requires immediate treatment by monitoring for the rapid onset of polyuria, polydipsia, weight loss, nausea, vomiting, dehydration, rapid respiration, weakness and clouding of sensorium, even coma
- EKGs may be useful for selected patients (e.g., those with personal or family history of QTc prolongation; cardiac arrhythmia; recent myocardial infarction; uncompensated heart failure; or taking agents that prolong QTc interval such as pimozide, thioridazine, selected antiarrhythmics, moxifloxacin, sparfloxacin, etc.)
- Patients at risk for electrolyte disturbances (e.g., patients on diuretic therapy) should have baseline and periodic serum potassium and magnesium measurements

SIDE EFFECTS

How Drug Causes Side Effects

- By blocking dopamine 2 receptors in the striatum, it can cause motor side effects, especially at high doses
- By blocking dopamine 2 receptors in the pituitary, it can cause elevations in prolactin
- Mechanism of weight gain and possible increased incidence of diabetes and dyslipidemia with atypical antipsychotics is unknown

Notable Side Effects

❋ Extrapyramidal symptoms
❋ Galactorrhea, amenorrhea
❋ Atypical antipsychotics may increase the risk for diabetes and dyslipidemia, although the specific risks associated with amisulpride are unknown
- Insomnia, sedation, agitation, anxiety
- Constipation, weight gain
- Rare tardive dyskinesia

 ### Life Threatening or Dangerous Side Effects

- Rare neuroleptic malignant syndrome
- Rare seizures
- Dose-dependent QTc prolongation
- Increased risk of death and cerebrovascular events in elderly patients with dementia-related psychosis

Weight Gain

unusual   not unusual   common   problematic

• Occurs in significant minority

Sedation

unusual   not unusual   common   problematic

• Many experience and/or can be significant in amount, especially at high doses

What To Do About Side Effects

• Wait
• Wait
• Wait
• Lower the dose
• For motor symptoms, add an anticholinergic agent
• Take more of the dose at bedtime to help reduce daytime sedation
• Weight loss, exercise programs, and medical management for high BMIs, diabetes, dyslipidemia
• Switch to another atypical antipsychotic

Best Augmenting Agents for Side Effects

• Benztropine or trihexyphenidyl for motor side effects
• Many side effects cannot be improved with an augmenting agent

DOSING AND USE

Usual Dosage Range

• Schizophrenia: 400–800 mg/day in 2 doses
• Negative symptoms only: 50–300 mg/day
• Dysthymia: 50 mg/day

Dosage Forms

• Different formulations may be available in different markets
• Tablet 50 mg, 100 mg, 200 mg, 400 mg
• Oral solution 100 mg/mL

How to Dose

• Initial 400–800 mg/day in 2 doses; daily doses above 400 mg should be divided in 2; maximum generally 1200 mg/day

 Dosing Tips

✳ Efficacy for negative symptoms in schizophrenia may be achieved at lower doses, while efficacy for positive symptoms may require higher doses
• Patients receiving low doses may only need to take the drug once daily
✳ For dysthymia and depression, use only low doses
✳ Dose-dependent QTc prolongation, so use with caution, especially at higher doses (>800 mg/day)
✳ Amisulpride may accumulate in patients with renal insufficiency, requiring lower dosing or switching to another antipsychotic to avoid QTc prolongation in these patients

Overdose

• Sedation, coma, hypotension, extrapyramidal symptoms

Long-Term Use

• Amisulpride is used for both acute and chronic schizophrenia treatment

Habit Forming

• No

How to Stop

• Slow down-titration (over 6 to 8 weeks), especially when simultaneously beginning a new antipsychotic while switching (i.e., cross-titration)
• Rapid discontinuation may lead to rebound psychosis and worsening of symptoms

Pharmacokinetics

• Elimination half-life approximately 12 hours
• Excreted largely unchanged

 Drug Interactions

• Can decrease the effects of levodopa, dopamine agonists
• Can increase the effects of antihypertensive drugs
• CNS effects may be increased if used with a CNS depressant
• May enhance QTc prolongation of other drugs capable of prolonging QTc interval

- Since amisulpride is only weakly metabolized, few drug interactions that could raise amisulpride plasma levels are expected

Other Warnings/ Precautions

- Use cautiously in patients with alcohol withdrawal or convulsive disorders because of possible lowering of seizure threshold
- If signs of neuroleptic malignant syndrome develop, treatment should be immediately discontinued
- Because amisulpride may dose-dependently prolong QTc interval, use with caution in patients who have bradycardia or who are taking drugs that can induce bradycardia (e.g., beta blockers, calcium channel blockers, clonidine, digitalis)
- Because amisulpride may dose-dependently prolong QTc interval, use with caution in patients who have hypokalemia and/or hypomagnesemia or who are taking drugs that can induce hypokalemia and/or magnesemia (e.g., diuretics, stimulant laxatives, intravenous amphotericin B, glucocorticoids, tetracosactide)
- Use only with caution if at all in Parkinson's disease or Lewy Body dementia, especially at high doses

Do Not Use

- If patient has pheochromocytoma
- If patient has prolactin-dependent tumor
- If patient is pregnant or nursing
- If patient is taking agents capable of significantly prolonging QTc interval (e.g., pimozide; thioridazine; selected antiarrhythmics such as quinidine, disopyramide, amiodarone, and sotalol; selected antibiotics such as moxifloxacin and sparfloxacin)
- If there is a history of QTc prolongation or cardiac arrhythmia, recent acute myocardial infarction, uncompensated heart failure
- If patient is taking cisapride, intravenous erythromycin, or pentamidine
- In children
- If there is a proven allergy to amisulpride

Renal Impairment

- Use with caution; drug may accumulate
- Amisulpride is eliminated by the renal route; in cases of severe renal insufficiency, the dose should be decreased and intermittent treatment or switching to another antipsychotic should be considered

Hepatic Impairment

- Use with caution, but dose adjustment not generally necessary

Cardiac Impairment

- Amisulpride produces a dose-dependent prolongation of QTc interval, which may be enhanced by the existence of bradycardia, hypokalemia, congenital or acquired long QTc interval, which should be evaluated prior to administering amisulpride
- Use with caution if treating concomitantly with a medication likely to produce prolonged bradycardia, hypokalemia, slowing of intracardiac conduction, or prolongation of the QTc interval
- Avoid amisulpride in patients with a known history of QTc prolongation, recent acute myocardial infarction, and uncompensated heart failure

Elderly

- Some patients may be more susceptible to sedative and hypotensive effects
- Although atypical antipsychotics are commonly used for behavioral disturbances in dementia, no agent has been approved for treatment of elderly patients with dementia-related psychosis
- Elderly patients with dementia-related psychosis treated with atypical antipsychotics are at an increased risk of death compared to placebo, and also have an increased risk of cerebrovascular events

 Children and Adolescents

- Efficacy and safety not established under age 18

 Pregnancy

- Although animal studies have not shown teratogenic effect, amisulpride is not recommended for use during pregnancy

- Psychotic symptoms may worsen during pregnancy and some form of treatment may be necessary
- Amisulpride may be preferable to anticonvulsant mood stabilizers if treatment is required during pregnancy

Breast Feeding

- Unknown if amisulpride is secreted in human breast milk, but all psychotropics assumed to be secreted in breast milk
- ✳ Recommended either to discontinue drug or bottle feed

THE ART OF PSYCHOPHARMACOLOGY

Potential Advantages

- Not as clearly associated with weight gain as some other atypical antipsychotics
- For patients who are responsive to low dose activation effects that reduce negative symptoms and depression

Potential Disadvantages

- Patients who have difficulty being compliant with twice daily dosing
- Patients for whom elevated prolactin may not be desired (e.g., possibly pregnant patients; pubescent girls with amenorrhea; postmenopausal women with low estrogen who do not take estrogen replacement therapy)
- Patients with severe renal impairment

Primary Target Symptoms

- Positive symptoms of psychosis
- Negative symptoms of psychosis
- Depressive symptoms

 Pearls

- ✳ Efficacy has been particularly well demonstrated in patients with predominantly negative symptoms
- ✳ The increase in prolactin caused by amisulpride may cause menstruation to stop
- Some treatment-resistant patients with inadequate responses to clozapine may benefit from amisulpride augmentation of clozapine
- Risks of diabetes and dyslipidemia not well studied, but does not seem to cause as

much weight gain as some other atypical antipsychotics
- Has atypical antipsychotic properties (i.e., antipsychotic action without a high incidence of extrapyramidal symptoms), especially at low doses, but not a serotonin dopamine antagonist
- Mediates its atypical antipsychotic properties via novel actions on dopamine receptors, perhaps dopamine stabilizing partial agonist actions on dopamine 2 receptors
- May be more of a dopamine 2 antagonist than aripiprazole, but less of a dopamine 2 antagonist than other atypical or conventional antipsychotics
- Low dose activating actions may be beneficial for negative symptoms in schizophrenia
- Very low doses may be useful in dysthymia
- Compared to sulpiride, amisulpride has better oral bioavailability and more potency, thus allowing lower dosing, less weight gain, and fewer extrapyramidal symptoms
- Compared to other atypical antipsychotics with potent serotonin 2A antagonism, amisulpride may have more extrapyramidal symptoms and prolactin elevation, but may still be classified as an atypical antipsychotic, particularly at low doses
- Patients have very similar antipsychotic responses to any conventional antipsychotic, which is different from atypical antipsychotics where antipsychotic responses of individual patients can occasionally vary greatly from one atypical antipsychotic to another
- Patients with inadequate responses to atypical antipsychotics may benefit from a trial of augmentation with a conventional antipsychotic or switching to a conventional antipsychotic
- However, long-term polypharmacy with a combination of a conventional antipsychotic with an atypical antipsychotic may combine their side effects without clearly augmenting the efficacy of either
- Although a frequent practice by some prescribers, adding two conventional antipsychotics together has little rationale and may reduce tolerability without clearly enhancing efficacy

Suggested Reading

Burns T, Bale R. Clinical advantages of amisulpride in the treatment of acute schizophrenia. J Int Med Res 2001; 29 (6): 451–66.

Curran MP, Perry CM. Spotlight on amisulpride in schizophrenia. CNS Drugs 2002; 16 (3): 207–11.

Leucht S, Pitschel-Walz G, Engel RR, Kissling W. Amisulpride, an unusual "atypical" antipsychotic: a meta-analysis of randomized controlled trials. Am J Psychiatry 2002; 159 (2): 180–90.

ARIPIPRAZOLE

THERAPEUTICS

Brands • Abilify
see index for additional brand names

Generic? Not in U.S., Europe, or Japan

Class
- Dopamine partial agonist (dopamine stabilizer, atypical antipsychotic, third generation antipsychotic; sometimes included as a second generation antipsychotic; also a mood stabilizer)

Commonly Prescribed For
(bold for FDA approved)
- **Schizophrenia**
- **Maintaining stability in schizophrenia**
- **Acute mania/mixed mania**
- **Bipolar maintenance**
- Bipolar depression
- Other psychotic disorders
- Behavioral disturbances in dementias
- Behavioral disturbances in children and adolescents
- Disorders associated with problems with impulse control

How The Drug Works
* Partial agonism at dopamine 2 receptors
- Theoretically reduces dopamine output when dopamine concentrations are high, thus improving positive symptoms and mediating antipsychotic actions
- Theoretically increases dopamine output when dopamine concentrations are low, thus improving cognitive, negative, and mood symptoms
- Actions at dopamine 3 receptors could theoretically contribute to aripiprazole's efficacy
- Partial agonism at 5HT1A receptors may be relevant at clinical doses
- Blockade of serotonin type 2A receptors may contribute at clinical doses to cause enhancement of dopamine release in certain brain regions, thus reducing motor side effects and possibly improving cognitive and affective symptoms

How Long Until It Works
- Psychotic and manic symptoms can improve within 1 week, but it may take several weeks for full effect on behavior as well as on cognition and affective stabilization
- Classically recommended to wait at least 4–6 weeks to determine efficacy of drug, but in practice some patients require up to 16–20 weeks to show a good response, especially on cognitive symptoms

If It Works
- Most often reduces positive symptoms in schizophrenia but does not eliminate them
- Can improve negative symptoms, as well as aggressive, cognitive, and affective symptoms in schizophrenia
- Most schizophrenic patients do not have a total remission of symptoms but rather a reduction of symptoms by about a third
- Perhaps 5–15% of schizophrenic patients can experience an overall improvement of greater than 50–60%, especially when receiving stable treatment for more than a year
- Such patients are considered super-responders or "awakeners" since they may be well enough to be employed, live independently, and sustain long-term relationships
- Many bipolar patients may experience a reduction of symptoms by half or more
- Continue treatment until reaching a plateau of improvement
- After reaching a satisfactory plateau, continue treatment for at least a year after first episode of psychosis
- For second and subsequent episodes of psychosis, treatment may need to be indefinite
- Even for first episodes of psychosis, it may be preferable to continue treatment indefinitely to avoid subsequent episodes
- Treatment may not only reduce mania but also prevent recurrences of mania in bipolar disorder

If It Doesn't Work
- Try one of the other atypical antipsychotics (risperidone, olanzapine, quetiapine, ziprasidone, amisulpride)
- If two or more antipsychotic monotherapies do not work, consider clozapine
- If no first-line atypical antipsychotic is effective, consider higher doses or augmentation with valproate or lamotrigine

- Some patients may require treatment with a conventional antipsychotic
- Consider noncompliance and switch to another antipsychotic with fewer side effects or to an antipsychotic that can be given by depot injection
- Consider initiating rehabilitation and psychotherapy
- Consider presence of concomitant drug abuse

 Best Augmenting Combos for Partial Response or Treatment-Resistance

- Valproic acid (valproate, divalproex, divalproex ER)
- Other mood stabilizing anticonvulsants (carbamazepine, oxcarbazepine, lamotrigine)
- Lithium
- Benzodiazepines

Tests

Before starting an atypical antipsychotic
✳ Weigh all patients and track BMI during treatment
- Get baseline personal and family history of diabetes, obesity, dyslipidemia, hypertension, and cardiovascular disease
✳ Get waist circumference (at umbilicus), blood pressure, fasting plasma glucose, and fasting lipid profile
- Determine if the patient is
  - overweight (BMI 25.0–29.9)
  - obese (BMI ≥30)
  - has pre-diabetes (fasting plasma glucose 100–125 mg/dl)
  - has diabetes (fasting plasma glucose >126 mg/dl)
  - has hypertension (BP >140/90 mm Hg)
  - has dyslipidemia (increased total cholesterol, LDL cholesterol, and triglycerides; decreased HDL cholesterol)
- Treat or refer such patients for treatment, including nutrition and weight management, physical activity counseling, smoking cessation, and medical management

Monitoring after starting an atypical antipsychotic
✳ BMI monthly for 3 months, then quarterly
✳ Blood pressure, fasting plasma glucose, fasting lipids within 3 months and then annually, but earlier and more frequently for patients with diabetes or who have gained >5% of initial weight
- Treat or refer for treatment and consider switching to another atypical antipsychotic for patients who become overweight, obese, pre-diabetic, diabetic, hypertensive, or dyslipidemic while receiving an atypical antipsychotic
✳ Even in patients without known diabetes, be vigilant for the rare but life threatening onset of diabetic ketoacidosis, which always requires immediate treatment, by monitoring for the rapid onset of polyuria, polydipsia, weight loss, nausea, vomiting, dehydration, rapid respiration, weakness and clouding of sensorium, even coma

SIDE EFFECTS

How Drug Causes Side Effects
- By blocking alpha 1 adrenergic receptors, it can cause dizziness, sedation, and hypotension
- Partial agonist actions at dopamine 2 receptors in the striatum can cause motor side effects, such as akathisia (occasionally)
- Partial agonist actions at dopamine 2 receptors can also cause nausea, occasional vomiting, and activating side effects
✳ Mechanism of any possible weight gain is unknown; weight gain is not common with aripiprazole and may thus have a different mechanism from atypical antipsychotics for which weight gain is common or problematic
✳ Mechanism of any possible increased incidence of diabetes or dyslipidemia is unknown; early experience suggests these complications are not clearly associated with aripiprazole and if present may therefore have a different mechanism from that of atypical antipsychotics associated with an increased incidence of diabetes and dyslipidemia

Notable Side Effects
✳ Dizziness, insomnia, akathisia, activation
✳ Nausea, vomiting
- Orthostatic hypotension, occasionally during initial dosing
- Constipation

- Headache, asthenia, sedation
- Theoretical risk of tardive dyskinesia

 ### Life Threatening or Dangerous Side Effects

- Rare neuroleptic malignant syndrome (much reduced risk compared to conventional antipsychotics)
- Rare seizures
- Increased risk of death and cerebrovascular events in elderly patients with dementia-related psychosis

Weight Gain

unusual — not unusual — common — problematic

- Reported in a few patients, especially those with low BMIs, but not expected
- Less frequent and less severe than for most other antipsychotics

Sedation

unusual — not unusual — common — problematic

- Reported in a few patients but not expected
- May be less than for some other antipsychotics, but never say never
- Can be activating

What To Do About Side Effects

- Wait
- Wait
- Wait
- Reduce the dose
- Anticholinergics may reduce akathisia when present
- Weight loss, exercise programs, and medical management for high BMIs, diabetes, dyslipidemia
- Switch to another atypical antipsychotic

Best Augmenting Agents for Side Effects

- Benztropine or trihexyphenidyl for motor side effects and akathisia
- Many side effects cannot be improved with an augmenting agent

DOSING AND USE

Usual Dosage Range

- 15–30 mg/day

Dosage Forms

- Tablet 5 mg, 10 mg, 15 mg, 20 mg, 30 mg
- Oral solution 1 mg/mL

How to Dose

- Initial approved recommendation is 10–15 mg/day; maximum approved dose 30 mg/day
- Oral solution: solution doses can be substituted for tablet doses on a mg-per-mg basis up to 25 mg; patients receiving 30 mg tablet should receive 25 mg solution

 ### Dosing Tips

- ✳ **For some, less may be more:** frequently, patients not acutely psychotic may need to be dosed lower (e.g., 2.5–10 mg/day) in order to avoid akathisia and activation and for maximum tolerability
- **For others, more may be more:** rarely, patients may need to be dosed higher than 30 mg/day for optimum efficacy
- Consider cutting 5 mg tablet in half (tablets not scored) or administering 1–5 mg as the oral solution for children and adolescents, as well as for adults very sensitive to side effects
- ✳ Although studies suggest patients switching to aripiprazole from another antipsychotic can do well with rapid switch or with cross-titration, clinical experience suggests many patients may do best by adding a full dose of aripiprazole to the maintenance dose of the first antipsychotic for at least several days and possibly as long as three or four weeks prior to slow down-titration of the first antipsychotic
- Rather than raise the dose above these levels in acutely agitated patients requiring acute antipsychotic actions, consider augmentation with a benzodiazepine or conventional antipsychotic, either orally or intramuscularly
- Rather than raise the dose above these levels in partial responders, consider augmentation with a mood stabilizing anticonvulsant, such as valproate or lamotrigine

- Children and elderly should generally be dosed at the lower end of the dosage spectrum
- Less expensive than some antipsychotics, more expensive than others depending on dose administered
- Due to its very long half-life, aripiprazole will take longer to reach steady state when initiating dosing, and longer to wash out when stopping dosing, than other atypical antipsychotics

Overdose
- No fatalities have been reported; sedation, vomiting

Long-Term Use
- Approved to delay relapse in long-term treatment of schizophrenia
- Approved for long-term maintenance in bipolar disorder
- Often used for long-term maintenance in various behavioral disorders

Habit Forming
- No

How to Stop
- Slow down-titration (over 6 to 8 weeks), especially when simultaneously beginning a new antipsychotic while switching (i.e., cross-titration)
- Rapid discontinuation could theoretically lead to rebound psychosis and worsening of symptoms

Pharmacokinetics
- Metabolized primarily by CYP450 2D6 and CYP450 3A4
- Mean elimination half-life 75 hours (aripiprazole) and 94 hours (major metabolite dehydro-aripiprazole)

 Drug Interactions
- Ketaconazole and possibly other CYP450 3A4 inhibitors such as nefazodone, fluvoxamine, and fluoxetine may increase plasma levels of aripiprazole
- Carbamazepine and possibly other inducers of CYP450 3A4 may decrease plasma levels of aripiprazole
- Quinidine and possibly other inhibitors of CYP450 2D6 such as paroxetine,

fluoxetine, and duloxetine may increase plasma levels of aripiprazole
- Aripiprazole may enhance the effects of antihypertensive drugs
- Aripiprazole may antagonize levodopa, dopamine agonists

 Other Warnings/ Precautions
- Use with caution in patients with conditions that predispose to hypotension (dehydration, overheating)
- Dysphagia has been associated with antipsychotic use, and aripiprazole should be used cautiously in patients at risk for aspiration pneumonia

Do Not Use
- If there is a proven allergy to aripiprazole

SPECIAL POPULATIONS

Renal Impairment
- Dose adjustment not necessary

Hepatic Impairment
- Dose adjustment not necessary

Cardiac Impairment
- Use in patients with cardiac impairment has not been studied, so use with caution because of risk of orthostatic hypotension

Elderly
- Dose adjustment generally not necessary, but some elderly patients may tolerate lower doses better
- Although atypical antipsychotics are commonly used for behavioral disturbances in dementia, no agent has been approved for treatment of elderly patients with dementia-related psychosis
- Elderly patients with dementia-related psychosis treated with atypical antipsychotics are at an increased risk of death compared to placebo, and also have an increased risk of cerebrovascular events

 Children and Adolescents
- Not officially recommended for patients under age 18

- Clinical experience and early data suggest aripiprazole may be safe and effective for behavioral disturbances in children and adolescents, especially at lower doses
- Children and adolescents using aripiprazole may need to be monitored more often than adults and may tolerate lower doses better

Pregnancy

- Risk Category C [some animal studies show adverse effects, no controlled studies in humans]
- Psychotic symptoms may worsen during pregnancy and some form of treatment may be necessary
- Aripiprazole may be preferable to anticonvulsant mood stabilizers if treatment is required during pregnancy

Breast Feeding

- Unknown if aripiprazole is secreted in human breast milk, but all psychotropics assumed to be secreted in breast milk
- ✳ Recommended either to discontinue drug or bottle feed
- Infants of women who choose to breast feed while on aripiprazole should be monitored for possible adverse effects

THE ART OF PSYCHOPHARMACOLOGY

Potential Advantages

- Some cases of psychosis and bipolar disorder refractory to treatment with other antipsychotics
- ✳ Patients concerned about gaining weight and patients who are already obese or overweight
- ✳ Patients with diabetes
- ✳ Patients with dyslipidemia (especially elevated triglycerides)
- Patients requiring rapid onset of antipsychotic action without dosage titration
- ✳ Patients who wish to avoid sedation

Potential Disadvantages

- Patients in whom sedation is desired
- May be more difficult to dose for children, elderly, or "off label" uses

Primary Target Symptoms

- Positive symptoms of psychosis
- Negative symptoms of psychosis
- Cognitive symptoms
- Unstable mood
- Aggressive symptoms

Pearls

- ✳ Well accepted in clinical practice when wanting to avoid weight gain because less weight gain than most other antipsychotics
- ✳ Well accepted in clinical practice when wanting to avoid sedation because less sedation than most other antipsychotics at all doses
- ✳ Can even be activating, which can be reduced by lowering the dose or starting at a lower dose
- If sedation is desired, a benzodiazepine can be added short-term at the initiation of treatment until symptoms of agitation and insomnia are stabilized or intermittently as needed
- A moderately priced atypical antipsychotic within the therapeutic dosing range
- ✳ May not have diabetes or dyslipidemia risk, but monitoring is still indicated
- Anecdotal reports of utility in treatment-resistant cases
- Has a very favorable tolerability profile in clinical practice
- Favorable tolerability profile leading to "off-label" uses for many indications other than schizophrenia (e.g., bipolar II disorder, including hypomanic, mixed, rapid cycling, and depressed phases; treatment-resistant depression; anxiety disorders)
- ✳ An intramuscular formulation is currently in development

Suggested Reading

Marder SR, McQuade RD, Stock E, Kaplita S, Marcus R, Safferman AZ, Saha A, Ali M, Iwamoto T. Aripiprazole in the treatment of schizophrenia: safety and tolerability in short-term, placebo-controlled trials. Schizophr Res 2003;61(2–3):123–36.

Sajatovic M. Treatment for mood and anxiety disorders: quetiapine and aripiprazole. Curr Psychiatry Rep 2003;5:320–6.

Shapiro DA, Renock S, Arrington E, Chiodo LA, Liu LX, Sibley DR, Roth BL, Mailman R. Aripiprazole, a novel atypical antipsychotic drug with a unique and robust pharmacology. Neuropsychopharmacology 2003;28:1400–11.

Stahl SM. Dopamine system stabilizers, aripiprazole, and the next generation of antipsychotics, part 1: "Goldilocks" actions at dopamine receptors. J Clin Psychiatry 2001;62:841–2.

Stahl SM. Dopamine system stabilizers, aripiprazole, and the next generation of antipsychotics, part 2: illustrating their mechanism of action. J Clin Psychiatry 2001;62 (12):923–4.

CARBAMAZEPINE

Brands • Tegretol
• Carbatrol
• Equetro
see index for additional brand names

Generic? Yes (not for extended release formulation)

Class

• Anticonvulsant, antineuralgic for chronic pain, voltage-sensitive sodium channel antagonist

Commonly Prescribed For
(bold for FDA approved)

• **Partial seizures with complex symptomatology**
• **Generalized tonic-clonic seizures (grand mal)**
• **Mixed seizure patterns**
• **Pain associated with true trigeminal neuralgia**
• **Acute mania/mixed mania (Equetro)**
• Glossopharyngeal neuralgia
• Bipolar depression
• Bipolar maintenance
• Psychosis, schizophrenia (adjunctive)

How The Drug Works

* Acts as a use-dependent blocker of voltage-sensitive sodium channels
* Interacts with the open channel conformation of voltage-sensitive sodium channels
* Interacts at a specific site of the alpha pore-forming subunit of voltage-sensitive sodium channels
• Inhibits release of glutamate

How Long Until It Works

• For acute mania, effects should occur within a few weeks
• May take several weeks to months to optimize an effect on mood stabilization
• Should reduce seizures by 2 weeks

If It Works

• The goal of treatment is complete remission of symptoms (e.g., seizures, mania, pain)

• Continue treatment until all symptoms are gone or until improvement is stable and then continue treating indefinitely as long as improvement persists
• Continue treatment indefinitely to avoid recurrence of mania and seizures
• Treatment of chronic neuropathic pain most often reduces but does not eliminate pain and is not a cure since symptoms usually recur after medicine stopped

If It Doesn't Work (for bipolar disorder)

* Many patients only have a partial response where some symptoms are improved but others persist or continue to wax and wane without stabilization of mood
• Other patients may be nonresponders, sometimes called treatment-resistant or treatment-refractory
• Consider increasing dose, switching to another agent or adding an appropriate augmenting agent
• Consider adding psychotherapy
• Consider biofeedback or hypnosis for pain
• For bipolar disorder, consider the presence of noncompliance and counsel patient
• Switch to another mood stabilizer with fewer side effects or to extended release carbamazepine
• Consider evaluation for another diagnosis or for a comorbid condition (e.g., medical illness, substance abuse, etc.)

Best Augmenting Combos for Partial Response or Treatment-Resistance

• Lithium
• Atypical antipsychotics (especially risperidone, olanzapine, quetiapine, ziprasidone, and aripiprazole)
• Valproate (carbamazepine can decrease valproate levels)
• Lamotrigine (carbamazepine can decrease lamotrigine levels)
* Antidepressants (with caution because antidepressants can destabilize mood in some patients, including induction of rapid cycling or suicidal ideation; in particular consider bupropion; also SSRIs, SNRIs, others; generally avoid TCAs, MAOIs)

Tests

❋ Before starting: blood count, liver, kidney, and thyroid function tests
• During treatment: blood count every 2 to 4 weeks for 2 months, then every 3 to 6 months throughout treatment
• During treatment: liver, kidney, and thyroid function tests every 6–12 months
• Consider monitoring sodium levels because of possibility of hyponatremia

SIDE EFFECTS

How Drug Causes Side Effects

• CNS side effects theoretically due to excessive actions at voltage-sensitive sodium channels
• Major metabolite (carbamazepine-10, 11 epoxide) may be the cause of many side effects
• Mild anticholinergic effects may contribute to sedation, blurred vision

Notable Side Effects

❋ Sedation, dizziness, confusion, unsteadiness, headache
❋ Nausea, vomiting, diarrhea
• Blurred vision
❋ Benign leukopenia (transient; in up to 10%)
❋ Rash

Life Threatening or Dangerous Side Effects

❋ Rare aplastic anemia, agranulocytosis (unusual bleeding or bruising, mouth sores, infections, fever, sore throat)
❋ Rare severe dermatologic reactions (Stevens Johnson syndrome)
• Rare cardiac problems
• Rare induction of psychosis or mania
❋ SIADH (syndrome of inappropriate antidiuretic hormone secretion) with hyponatremia
• Increased frequency of generalized convulsions (in patients with atypical absence seizures)

Weight Gain

unusual   not unusual   common   problematic

• Occurs in significant minority

Sedation

unusual   not unusual   common   problematic

• Frequent and can be significant in amount
• Some patients may not tolerate it
• Dose-related
• Can wear off with time, but commonly does not wear off at high doses
• CNS side effects significantly lower with controlled release formulation (e.g., Equetro, Carbatrol)

What To Do About Side Effects

• Wait
• Wait
• Wait
• Take with food or split dose to avoid gastrointestinal effects
• Extended release carbamazepine can be sprinkled on soft food
• Take at night to reduce daytime sedation
• Switch to another agent or to extended release carbamazepine

Best Augmenting Agents for Side Effects

• Many side effects cannot be improved with an augmenting agent

DOSING AND USE

Usual Dosage Range

• 400–1200 mg/day
• Under age 6: 10–20 mg/kg/day

Dosage Forms

• Tablet 100 mg chewable, 200 mg chewable, 200 mg
• Extended release tablet 100 mg, 200 mg, 400 mg
• Extended release capsule 100 mg, 200 mg, 300 mg
• Oral suspension 100 mg/5mL (450 mL)

How to Dose

• For bipolar disorder and seizures (ages 13 and older): initial 200 mg twice daily (tablet) or 1 teaspoon (100 mg) 4 times a day (suspension); each week increase by up to 200 mg/day in divided doses (2 doses for extended release formulation, 3–4 doses for other tablets); maximum dose generally 1200 mg/day for adults and

1000 mg/day for children under age 15; maintenance dose generally 800–1200 mg/day for adults; some patients may require up to 1600 mg/day
- Seizures (under age 13): see Children and Adolescents
- Trigeminal neuralgia: initial 100 mg twice daily (tablet) or 0.5 teaspoon (50 mg) 4 times a day; each week increase by up to 200 mg/day in divided doses (100 mg every 12 hours for tablet formulations, 50 mg 4 times a day for suspension formulation); maximum dose generally 1200 mg/day
- Lower initial dose and slower titration should be used for carbamazepine suspension

 Dosing Tips

- Higher peak levels occur with the suspension formulation than with the same dose of the tablet formulation, so suspension should generally be started at a lower dose and titrated slowly
- Take carbamazepine with food to avoid gastrointestinal effects
- ✳ Slow dose titration may delay onset of therapeutic action but enhance tolerability to sedating side effects
- Controlled release formulations (e.g., Equetro, Carbatrol) can significantly reduce sedation and other CNS side effects
- Should titrate slowly in the presence of other sedating agents, such as other anticonvulsants, in order to best tolerate additive sedative side effects
- ✳ Can sometimes minimize the impact of carbamazepine upon the bone marrow by dosing slowly and monitoring closely when initiating treatment; initial trend to leukopenia/neutropenia may reverse with continued conservative dosing over time and allow subsequent dosage increases with careful monitoring
- ✳ Carbamazepine often requires a dosage adjustment upward with time, as the drug induces its own metabolism, thus lowering its own plasma levels over the first several weeks to months of treatment
- Do not break or chew carbamazepine extended release tablets as this will alter controlled release properties

Overdose
- Can be fatal (lowest known fatal dose in adults is 3.2 g, in adolescents is 4 g, and in children is 1.6 g); nausea, vomiting, involuntary movements, irregular heartbeat, urinary retention, trouble breathing, sedation, coma

Long-Term Use
- May lower sex drive
- Monitoring of liver, kidney, thyroid functions, blood counts and sodium may be required

Habit Forming
- No

How to Stop
- Taper; may need to adjust dosage of concurrent medications as carbamazepine is being discontinued
- ✳ Rapid discontinuation may increase the risk of relapse in bipolar disorder
- Epilepsy patients may seize upon withdrawal, especially if withdrawal is abrupt
- Discontinuation symptoms uncommon

Pharmacokinetics
- Metabolized in the liver, primarily by CYP450 3A4
- Renally excreted
- Active metabolite (carbamazepine-10,11 epoxide)
- Initial half-life 26–65 hours (35–40 hours for extended release formulation); half-life 12–17 hours with repeated doses
- Half-life of active metabolite is approximately 34 hours
- ✳ Is not only a substrate for CYP450 3A4, but also an inducer of CYP450 3A4
- ✳ Thus, carbamazepine induces its own metabolism, often requiring an upward dosage adjustment

 Drug Interactions

- Enzyme-inducing antiepileptic drugs (carbamazepine itself as well as phenobarbital, phenytoin, and primidone) may increase the clearance of carbamazepine and lower its plasma levels
- CYP450 3A4 inducers, such as carbamazepine itself, can lower the plasma levels of carbamazepine

- CYP450 3A4 inhibitors, such as nefazodone, fluvoxamine, and fluoxetine, can increase plasma levels of carbamazepine
- Carbamazepine can increase plasma levels of clomipramine, phenytoin, primidone
- Carbamazepine can decrease plasma levels of acetaminophen, clozapine, benzodiazepines, dicumarol, doxycycline, theophylline, warfarin, and haloperidol as well as other anticonvulsants such as phensuximide, methsuximide, ethosuximide, phenytoin, tiagabine, topiramate, lamotrigine, and valproate
- Carbamazepine can decrease plasma levels of hormonal contraceptives and adversely affect their efficacy
- Combined use of carbamazepine with other anticonvulsants may lead to altered thyroid function
- Combined use of carbamazepine and lithium may increase risk of neurotoxic effects
- Depressive effects are increased by other CNS depressants (alcohol, MAOIs, other anticonvulsants, etc.)
- Combined use of carbamazepine suspension with liquid formulations of chlorpromazine has been shown to result in excretion of an orange rubbery precipitate; because of this, combined use of carbamazepine suspension with any liquid medicine is not recommended

 Other Warnings/ Precautions

❋ Patients should be monitored carefully for signs of unusual bleeding or bruising, mouth sores, infections, fever, or sore throat, as the risk of aplastic anemia and agranulocytosis with carbamazepine use is 5–8 times greater than in the general population (risk in the untreated general population is 6 patients per one million per year for agranulocytosis and 2 patients per one million per year for aplastic anemia)
- Because carbamazepine has a tricyclic chemical structure, it is not recommended to be taken with MAOIs, including 14 days after MAOIs are stopped; do not start an MAOI until 2 weeks after discontinuing carbamazepine
- May exacerbate narrow angle-closure glaucoma

- Because carbamazepine can lower plasma levels of hormonal contraceptives, it may also reduce their effectiveness
- May need to restrict fluid intake because of risk of developing syndrome of inappropriate antidiuretic hormone secretion, hyponatremia and its complications
- Use with caution in patients with mixed seizure disorders that include atypical absence seizures because carbamazepine has been associated with increased frequency of generalized convulsions in such patients

Do Not Use
- If patient is taking an MAOI
- If patient has history of bone marrow suppression
- If there is a proven allergy to any tricyclic compound
- If there is a proven allergy to carbamazepine

SPECIAL POPULATIONS

Renal Impairment
- Carbamazepine is renally secreted, so the dose may need to be lowered

Hepatic Impairment
- Drug should be used with caution
- Rare cases of hepatic failure have occurred

Cardiac Impairment
- Drug should be used with caution

Elderly
- Some patients may tolerate lower doses better
- Elderly patients may be more susceptible to adverse effects

 Children and Adolescents
- Approved use for epilepsy; therapeutic range of total carbamazepine in plasma is considered the same for children and adults
- Ages 6–12: initial dose 100 mg twice daily (tablets) or 0.5 teaspoon (50 mg) 4 times a day (suspension); each week increase by up to 100 mg/day in divided doses (2

doses for extended release formulation, 3–4 doses for all other formulations); maximum dose generally 1000 mg/day; maintenance dose generally 400–800 mg/day
- Ages 5 and younger: initial 10–20 mg/kg/day in divided doses (2–3 doses for tablet formulations, 4 doses for suspension); increase weekly as needed; maximum dose generally 35 mg/kg/day

 Pregnancy
- Risk category D [positive evidence of risk to human fetus; potential benefits may still justify its use during pregnancy]
- ✴ Use during first trimester may raise risk of neural tube defects (e.g., spina bifida) or other congenital anomalies
- Use in women of childbearing potential requires weighing potential benefits to the mother against the risks to the fetus
- ✴ If drug is continued, perform tests to detect birth defects
- ✴ If drug is continued, start on folate 1 mg/day early in pregnancy to reduce risk of neural tube defects
- Antiepileptic Drug Pregnancy Registry: (888) 233-2334
- Use of anticonvulsants in combination may cause a higher prevalence of teratogenic effects than anticonvulsant monotherapy
- Taper drug if discontinuing
- Seizures, even mild seizures, may cause harm to the embryo/fetus
- ✴ For bipolar patients, carbamazepine should generally be discontinued before anticipated pregnancies
- Recurrent bipolar illness during pregnancy can be quite disruptive
- For bipolar patients, given the risk of relapse in the postpartum period, some form of mood stabilizer treatment may need to be restarted immediately after delivery if patient is unmedicated during pregnancy
- ✴ Atypical antipsychotics may be preferable to lithium or anticonvulsants such as carbamazepine if treatment of bipolar disorder is required during pregnancy
- Bipolar symptoms may recur or worsen during pregnancy and some form of treatment may be necessary

Breast Feeding
- Some drug is found in mother's breast milk
- ✴ Recommended either to discontinue drug or bottle feed
- If drug is continued while breast feeding, infant should be monitored for possible adverse effects, including hematological effects
- If infant shows signs of irritability or sedation, drug may need to be discontinued
- Some cases of neonatal seizures, respiratory depression, vomiting, and diarrhea have been reported in infants whose mothers received carbamazepine during pregnancy
- ✴ Bipolar disorder may recur during the postpartum period, particularly if there is a history of prior postpartum episodes of either depression or psychosis
- Relapse rates may be lower in women who receive prophylactic treatment for postpartum episodes of bipolar disorder
- Atypical antipsychotics and anticonvulsants such as valproate may be safer than carbamazepine during the postpartum period when breast feeding

THE ART OF PSYCHOPHARMACOLOGY

Potential Advantages
- Treatment-resistant bipolar and psychotic disorders

Potential Disadvantages
- Patients who do not wish to or cannot comply with blood testing and close monitoring
- Patients who cannot tolerate sedation
- Pregnant patients

Primary Target Symptoms
- Incidence of seizures
- Unstable mood, especially mania
- Pain

 Pearls
- Carbamazepine was the first anticonvulsant widely used for the treatment of bipolar disorder and is now formally approved for acute mania and mixed mania

✳ An extended release formulation has better evidence of efficacy and improved tolerability in bipolar disorder than does immediate release carbamazepine
• Dosage frequency as well as sedation, diplopia, confusion, and ataxia may be reduced with extended release carbamazepine
• Risk of serious side effects is greatest in the first few months of treatment

• Common side effects such as sedation often abate after a few months
✳ May be effective in patients who fail to respond to lithium or other mood stabilizers
• May be effective for the depressed phase of bipolar disorder and for maintenance in bipolar disorder
• Can be complicated to use with concomitant medications

Suggested Reading

Brambilla P, Barale F, Soares JC. Perspectives on the use of anticonvulsants in the treatment of bipolar disorder. Int J Neuropsychopharmacol. 2001; 4: 421–46.

Leucht S, McGrath J, White P, Kissling W. Carbamazepine for schizophrenia and schizoaffective psychoses. Cochrane Database Syst Rev. 2002;(3):CD001258.

Marson AG, Williamson PR, Hutton JL, Clough HE, Chadwick DW. Carbamazepine versus valproate monotherapy for epilepsy. Cochrane Database Syst Rev. 2000; (3): CD001030.

Weisler RH, Kalali AH, Ketter TA. A multicenter, randomized, double-blind, placebo-controlled trial of extended-release carbamazepine capsules as monotherapy for bipolar disorder patients with manic or mixed episodes. J Clin Psychiatry 2004; 65: 478–84.

THERAPEUTICS

Brands • Clozaril
• Leponex
see index for additional brand names

Generic? Yes

Class

• Atypical antipsychotic (serotonin-dopamine antagonist; second generation antipsychotic; also a mood stabilizer)

Commonly Prescribed For
(bold for FDA approved)

• **Treatment-resistant schizophrenia**
• **Reduction in risk of recurrent suicidal behavior in patients with schizophrenia or schizoaffective disorder**
• Treatment-resistant bipolar disorder
• Violent aggressive patients with psychosis and other brain disorders not responsive to other treatments

How The Drug Works

• Blocks dopamine 2 receptors, reducing positive symptoms of psychosis and stabilizing affective symptoms
• Blocks serotonin 2A receptors, causing enhancement of dopamine release in certain brain regions and thus reducing motor side effects and possibly improving cognitive and affective symptoms
• Interactions at a myriad of other neurotransmitter receptors may contribute to clozapine's efficacy
✳ Specifically, interactions at 5HT2C and 5HT1A receptors may contribute to efficacy for cognitive and affective symptoms in some patients
• Mechanism of efficacy for psychotic patients who do not respond to conventional antipsychotics is unknown

How Long Until It Works

• Psychotic and manic symptoms can improve within 1 week, especially with first-line use, but often takes several weeks for full effect on behavior as well as on cognition and affective stabilization, especially in treatment-resistant cases
• Classically recommended to wait at least 4–6 weeks to determine efficacy of drug, but in practice patients often require up to 16–20 weeks to show a good response, especially in treatment-resistant cases

If It Works

• As for other antipsychotics, most often reduces positive symptoms in schizophrenia but does not eliminate them
✳ However, clozapine may reduce positive symptoms in patients who do not respond to other antipsychotics, especially other conventional antipsychotics
• Can improve negative symptoms, as well as aggressive, cognitive, and affective symptoms in schizophrenia
• Most schizophrenic patients do not have a total remission of symptoms but rather a reduction of symptoms by about a third
• Many patients with bipolar disorder and other disorders with psychotic, aggressive, violent, impulsive, and other types of behavioral disturbances may respond to clozapine when other agents have failed
• Perhaps 5–15% of schizophrenic patients can experience an overall improvement of greater than 50–60%, especially when receiving stable treatment for more than a year
✳ Such patients are considered super-responders or "awakeners" since they may be well enough to be employed, live independently, and sustain long-term relationships; super-responders are anecdotally reported more often with clozapine than with some other antipsychotics
• Continue treatment until reaching a plateau of improvement
• After reaching a satisfactory plateau, continue treatment for at least a year after first episode of psychosis
• For second and subsequent episodes of psychosis, treatment may need to be indefinite
• Even for first episodes of psychosis, it may be preferable to continue treatment indefinitely to avoid subsequent episodes
• Treatment may not only reduce mania but also prevent recurrences of mania in bipolar disorder

If It Doesn't Work

• Some patients may respond better if switched to a conventional antipsychotic

✳ Some patients may require augmentation with a conventional antipsychotic or with an atypical antipsychotic (especially risperidone or amisulpride), but these are the most refractory of all psychotic patients and such treatment is very expensive

✳ Consider augmentation with valproate or lamotrigine

• Consider noncompliance and switch to another antipsychotic with fewer side effects or to an antipsychotic that can be given by depot injection

• Consider initiating rehabilitation and psychotherapy

• Consider presence of concomitant drug abuse

Best Augmenting Combos for Partial Response or Treatment-Resistance

• Valproic acid (valproate, divalproex, divalproex ER)
• Lamotrigine
• Other mood stabilizing anticonvulsants (carbamazepine, oxcarbazepine)
• Conventional antipsychotics
• Benzodiazepines
• Lithium

Tests

✳ Complete blood count before treatment, weekly for 6 months of treatment, biweekly for months 6–12, and every 4 weeks thereafter

• Weekly monitoring of white blood cell count and absolute neurotrophil count for a period of 12 months is required in patients who are rechallenged with clozapine after recovery from an initial episode of moderate leukopenia (white blood cell count between 2000/mm³ and 3000/mm³, absolute neutrophil count between 1000/mm³ and 1500/mm³)

Before starting an atypical antipsychotic

✳ Weigh all patients and track BMI during treatment

• Get baseline personal and family history of diabetes, obesity, dyslipidemia, hypertension, and cardiovascular disease

✳ Get waist circumference (at umbilicus), blood pressure, fasting plasma glucose, and fasting lipid profile

• Determine if the patient is
  • overweight (BMI 25.0–29.9)
  • obese (BMI ≥30)
  • has pre-diabetes (fasting plasma glucose 100–125 mg/dl)
  • has diabetes (fasting plasma glucose >126 mg/dl)
  • has hypertension (BP >140/90 mm Hg)
  • has dyslipidemia (increased total cholesterol, LDL cholesterol, and triglycerides; decreased HDL cholesterol)

• Treat or refer such patients for treatment, including nutrition and weight management, physical activity counseling, smoking cessation, and medical management

Monitoring after starting an atypical antipsychotic

✳ BMI monthly for 3 months, then quarterly

✳ Blood pressure, fasting plasma glucose, fasting lipids within 3 months and then annually, but earlier and more frequently for patients with diabetes or who have gained >5% of initial weight

• Treat or refer for treatment and consider switching to another atypical antipsychotic for patients who become overweight, obese, pre-diabetic, diabetic, hypertensive, or dyslipidemic while receiving an atypical antipsychotic

✳ Even in patients without known diabetes, be vigilant for the rare but life threatening onset of diabetic ketoacidosis, which always requires immediate treatment, by monitoring for the rapid onset of polyuria, polydipsia, weight loss, nausea, vomiting, dehydration, rapid respiration, weakness and clouding of sensorium, even coma

• Liver function testing, electrocardiogram, general physical exam, and assessment of baseline cardiac status before starting treatment

• Liver tests may be necessary during treatment in patients who develop nausea, vomiting, or anorexia

✳ Electrocardiograms and cardiac evaluation to rule out myocarditis may be necessary during treatment in patients who develop shortness of breath or chest pain

SIDE EFFECTS

How Drug Causes Side Effects
- By blocking histamine 1 receptors in the brain, it can cause sedation and possibly weight gain
- By blocking alpha 1 adrenergic receptors, it can cause dizziness, sedation, and hypotension
- By blocking muscarinic 1 receptors, it can cause dry mouth, constipation, and sedation
- By blocking dopamine 2 receptors in the striatum, it can cause motor side effects (very rare)
- Mechanism of weight gain and increased incidence of diabetes and dyslipidemia with atypical antipsychotics is unknown but insulin regulation may be impaired by blocking pancreatic M3 muscarinic receptors

Notable Side Effects
- ✳ Probably increases risk for diabetes and dyslipidemia
- ✳ Increased salivation (can be severe)
- ✳ Sweating
- Dizziness, sedation, headache, tachycardia, hypotension
- Nausea, constipation, dry mouth, weight gain
- Rare tardive dyskinesia (no reports have directly implicated clozapine in the development of tardive dyskinesia)

Life Threatening or Dangerous Side Effects
- Hyperglycemia, in some cases extreme and associated with ketoacidosis or hyperosmolar coma or death, has been reported in patients taking atypical antipsychotics
- Agranulocytosis (includes flu-like symptoms or signs of infection)
- Seizures (risk increases with dose)
- Neuroleptic malignant syndrome (more likely when clozapine is used with another agent)
- Pulmonary embolism (may include deep vein thrombosis or respiratory symptoms)
- Myocarditis
- Increased risk of death and cerebrovascular events in elderly patients with dementia-related psychosis

Weight Gain

unusual   not unusual   common   problematic

- Frequent and can be significant in amount
- Can become a health problem in some
- More than for some other antipsychotics, but never say always as not a problem in everyone

Sedation

unusual   not unusual   common   problematic

- Frequent and can be significant in amount
- Some patients may not tolerate it
- More than for some other antipsychotics, but never say always as not a problem in everyone
- Can wear off over time
- Can reemerge as dose increases and then wear off again over time

What To Do About Side Effects
- Patients must inform prescriber immediately of any flu-like symptoms, muscle rigidity, altered mental status, irregular pulse or blood pressure
- Take at bedtime to help reduce daytime sedation
- Sedation may wear off with time
- Start dosing low and increase slowly as side effects wear off at each dosing increment
- Weight loss, exercise programs, and medical management for high BMIs, diabetes, dyslipidemia
- Switch to another agent

Best Augmenting Agents for Side Effects
- Many side effects cannot be improved with an augmenting agent

DOSING AND USE

Usual Dosage Range
- 300–450 mg/day

Dosage Forms
- Tablet 12.5 mg, 25 mg scored, 50 mg, 100 mg scored
- Orally disintegrating tablet 25 mg, 50 mg, 100 mg

How to Dose

- Initial 25 mg in 2 divided doses; increase by 25–50 mg/day each day until desired efficacy is reached; maintenance dose 300–450 mg/day; doses above 300 mg/day should be divided; increases in doses above 450 mg/day should be made weekly; maximum dose generally 900 mg/day

Dosing Tips

- Prescriptions are generally given 1 week at a time for the first 6 months of treatment because of the risk of agranulocytosis; for months 6–12 prescriptions can generally be given 2 weeks at a time; after 12 months prescriptions can generally be given monthly
- ✱ Treatment should be suspended if absolute neutrophil count falls below 1,000/mm^3
- Treatment should be suspended if white blood cell count falls below 2,000/mm^3
- Treatment should be suspended if eosinophil count rises above 4,000/mm^3, and continued once it falls below 3,000/mm^3
- If treatment is discontinued for more than 2 days, it may need to be reinitiated at a lower dose and slowly increased in order to maximize tolerability
- Plasma half-life suggests twice daily administration, but in practice it may be given once a day at night
- Doses over 550 mg/day may require concomitant anticonvulsant administration to reduce the chances of a seizure
- ✱ Rebound psychosis may occur unless dose is very slowly tapered, by 100 mg/week or less

Overdose

- Sometimes lethal; changes in heart rhythm, excess salivation, respiratory depression, altered state of consciousness

Long-Term Use

- Treatment to reduce risk of suicidal behavior should be continued for at least 2 years
- Often used for long-term maintenance in treatment-resistant schizophrenia

Habit Forming

- No

How to Stop

- Slow down-titration (over 6 to 8 weeks), especially when simultaneously beginning a new antipsychotic while switching (i.e., cross-titration)
- Blood testing is necessary every week for 4 weeks following discontinuation, or until WBC ≥3,500/mm^3 and ANC ≥2,000/mm^3
- ✱ Rapid discontinuation may lead to rebound psychosis and worsening of symptoms

Pharmacokinetics

- Half-life 5–16 hours
- Metabolized by multiple CYP450 enzymes, including 1A2, 2D6, and 3A4

Drug Interactions

- Dose may need to be reduced if given in conjunction with CYP450 1A2 inhibitors (e.g., fluvoxamine)
- Dose may need to be raised if given in conjunction with CYP450 1A2 inducers (e.g., cigarette smoke)
- CYP450 2D6 inhibitors (e.g., paroxetine, fluoxetine, duloxetine) can raise clozapine levels, but dosage adjustment usually not necessary
- CYP450 3A4 inhibitors (e.g., nefazodone, fluvoxamine, fluoxetine) can raise clozapine levels, but dosage adjustment usually not necessary
- Clozapine may enhance effects of antihypertensive drugs

Other Warnings/ Precautions

- Possible association between myocarditis and cardiomyopathy and clozapine use, even in physically healthy individuals
- Should not be used in conjunction with agents that are known to cause agranulocytosis
- Use with caution in patients with glaucoma
- Use with caution in patients with enlarged prostate

Do Not Use

- In patients with myeloproliferative disorder
- In patients with uncontrolled epilepsy
- In patients with granulocytopenia
- In patients with CNS depression
- If there is a proven allergy to clozapine

SPECIAL POPULATIONS

Renal Impairment
• Should be used with caution

Hepatic Impairment
• Should be used with caution

Cardiac Impairment
• Should be used with caution, particularly if patient is taking concomitant medication

Elderly
• Some patients may tolerate lower doses better
• Although atypical antipsychotics are commonly used for behavioral disturbances in dementia, no agent has been approved for treatment of elderly patients with dementia-related psychosis
• Elderly patients with dementia-related psychosis treated with atypical antipsychotics are at an increased risk of death compared to placebo, and also have an increased risk of cerebrovascular events

 Children and Adolescents
• Safety and efficacy have not been established
• Preliminary research has suggested efficacy in early-onset treatment-resistant schizophrenia
• Children and adolescents taking clozapine should be monitored more often than adults

Pregnancy
• Risk Category B [animal studies do not show adverse effects, no controlled studies in humans]
• Psychotic symptoms may worsen during pregnancy and some form of treatment may be necessary
• Clozapine should be used only when the potential benefits outweigh potential risks to the fetus

Breast Feeding
• Unknown if clozapine is secreted in human breast milk, but all psychotropics assumed to be secreted in breast milk
✳ Recommended either to discontinue drug or bottle feed

• Infants of women who choose to breast feed while on clozapine should be monitored for possible adverse effects

THE ART OF PSYCHOPHARMACOLOGY

Potential Advantages
✳ Treatment-resistant schizophrenia
✳ Violent, aggressive patients
✳ Patients with tardive dyskinesia
✳ Patients with suicidal behavior

Potential Disadvantages
✳ Patients with diabetes, obesity, and/or dyslipidemia
• Patients with cardiac impairment

Primary Target Symptoms
• Positive symptoms of psychosis
• Negative symptoms of psychosis
• Cognitive symptoms
• Affective symptoms
• Suicidal behavior
• Violence and aggression

 Pearls
✳ Not a first-line treatment choice in most countries
✳ Most efficacious but most dangerous
✳ Documented efficacy in treatment-refractory schizophrenia
• May reduce violence and aggression in difficult cases, including forensic cases
✳ Reduces suicide in schizophrenia
• May reduce substance abuse
• May improve tardive dyskinesia
• Little or no prolactin elevation, motor side effects, or tardive dyskinesia
• Clinical improvements often continue slowly over several years
• Cigarette smoke can decrease clozapine levels and patients may be at risk for relapse if they begin or increase smoking
• More weight gain than many other antipsychotics – does not mean every patient gains weight

Suggested Reading

Iqbal MM, Rahman A, Husain Z, Mahmud SZ, Ryan WG, Feldman JM. Clozapine: a clinical review of adverse effects and management. Ann Clin Psychiatry 2003;15:33–48.

Lieberman JA. Maximizing clozapine therapy: managing side effects. J Clin Psychiatry 1998;59 (suppl 3):38–43.

Schulte P. What is an adequate trial with clozapine?: therapeutic drug monitoring and time to response in treatment-refractory schizophrenia. Clin Pharmacokinet 2003;42:607–18.

Wagstaff A, Perry C. Clozapine: in prevention of suicide in patients with schizophrenia or schizoaffective disorder. CNS Drugs 2003;17:273–80

Wahlbeck K, Cheine M, Essali A, Adams C. Evidence of clozapine's effectiveness in schizophrenia: a systematic review and meta-analysis of randomized trials. Am J Psychiatry 1999;156:990–999.

Brands • Tercian
see index for additional brand names

Generic? Not in the U.S.

Class

• Conventional antipsychotic (neuroleptic, phenothiazine, dopamine 2 antagonist, serotonin dopamine antagonist)

Commonly Prescribed For
(bold for FDA approved)

• Schizophrenia
✳ Anxiety associated with psychosis (short-term)
• Anxiety associated with nonpsychotic disorders, including mood disorders and personality disorders (short-term)
• Severe depression
• Bipolar disorder
• Other psychotic disorders
• Acute agitation/aggression (injection)
• Benzodiazepine withdrawal

How The Drug Works

• Blocks dopamine 2 receptors, reducing positive symptoms of psychosis
✳ Although classified as a conventional antipsychotic, cyamemazine is a potent serotonin 2A antagonist
• Affinity at a myriad of other neurotransmitter receptors may contribute to cyamemazine's efficacy
✳ Specifically, antagonist actions at 5HT2C receptors may contribute to notable anxiolytic effects in many patients
• 5HT2C antagonist actions may also contribute to antidepressant actions in severe depression and to improvement of cognitive and negative symptoms of schizophrenia in some patients

How Long Until It Works

• Psychotic symptoms can improve with high doses within 1 week, but it may take several weeks for full effect on behavior
• Anxiolytic actions can improve with low doses within 1 week, but it may take several days to weeks for full effect on behavior

If It Works

• High doses most often reduce positive symptoms in schizophrenia but do not eliminate them
• Low doses most often reduce anxiety symptoms in psychotic and nonpsychotic disorders
• Most schizophrenia patients do not have a total remission of symptoms but rather a reduction of symptoms by about a third
• Continue treatment in schizophrenia until reaching a plateau of improvement
• After reaching a satisfactory plateau, continue treatment for at least a year, after first episode of psychosis in schizophrenia
• For second and subsequent episodes of psychosis in schizophrenia, treatment may need to be indefinite
• For symptomatic treatment of anxiety in psychotic and nonpsychotic disorders, treatment may also need to be indefinite while monitoring the risks versus the benefits of long term treatment
• Reduces symptoms of acute psychotic mania but not proven as a mood stabilizer or as an effective maintenance treatment in bipolar disorder
• After reducing acute psychotic symptoms in mania, consider switching to a mood stabilizer and/or an atypical antipsychotic for long term mood stabilization and maintenance

If It Doesn't Work

• For treatment of psychotic symptoms, consider trying one of the first line atypical antipsychotics (risperidone, olanzapine, quetiapine, ziprasidone, aripiprazole, amisulpiride)
• Consider trying another conventional antipsychotic
• If 2 or more antipsychotic monotherapies do not work, consider clozapine
• For treatment of anxiety symptoms, consider adding a benzodiazepine or switching to a benzodiazepine

Best Augmenting Combos for Partial Response or Treatment-Resistance

• Generally, best to switch to another agent
• Augmentation of conventional antipsychotics has not been systematically studied

- Addition of a mood stabilizing anticonvulsant such as valproate, carbamazepine, or lamotrigine may be helpful in both schizophrenia and bipolar mania
- Augmentation with lithium in bipolar mania may be helpful
- Addition of a benzodiazepine, especially for short term agitation
- Addition of antidepressants for severe depression

Tests

✻ Since conventional antipsychotics are frequently associated with weight gain, before starting treatment, weigh all patients and determine if the patient is already overweight (BMI 25.0–29.9) or obese BMI ≥30)
- Before giving a drug that can cause weight gain to an overweight or obese patient, consider determining whether the patient already has pre-diabetes (fasting glucose 100–125 mg/dl), diabetes (fasting plasma glucose >125 mg/dl) or dyslipidemia (increased total cholesterol, LDL cholesterol and triglycerides; decreased HDL cholesterol), and treat or refer such patients for treatment, including nutrition and weight management, physical activity counseling, smoking cessation and medical management
✻ Monitor weight, and BMI during treatment
✻ While giving a drug to a patient who has gained >5% of initial weight, consider evaluating for the presence of pre-diabetes, diabetes or dyslipidemia, or consider switching to a different antipsychotic
- Should check blood pressure in the elderly before starting and for the first few weeks of treatment
- Monitoring elevated prolactin levels of dubious clinical benefit

SIDE EFFECTS

How Drug Causes Side Effects

- By blocking dopamine 2 receptors in the striatum, it can cause motor side effects at antipsychotic (high) doses
- Much lower propensity to cause motor side effects at low doses used to treat anxiety

- By blocking dopamine 2 receptors in the pituitary, it can cause elevations in prolactin, but unlike other conventional antipsychotics, prolactin elevations at low doses of cyamemazine are uncommon or transient
- By blocking dopamine 2 receptors excessively in the mesocortical and mesolimbic dopamine pathways, especially at high doses, it can cause worsening of negative and cognitive symptoms (neuroleptic-induced deficit syndrome)
- Anticholinergic actions, especially at high doses, may cause sedation, blurred vision, constipation, dry mouth
- Antihistamine actions may contribute to anxiolytic actions at low doses and to sedation and weight gain at high doses
- By blocking alpha 1 adrenergic receptors, cyamemazine can cause dizziness, sedation and hypotension especially at high doses
- Mechanism of weight gain and any possible increased incidence of diabetes and dyslipidemia with conventional antipsychotics is unknown

Notable Side Effects

✻ Neuroleptic induced deficit syndrome (unusual at low doses)
- Akathisia
- Extrapyramidal symptoms, Parkinsonism, tardive dyskinesia (unusual at low doses)
- Galactorrhea, amenorrhea (unusual at low doses)
- Hypotension, tachycardia (unusual at low doses)
- Dry mouth, constipation, vision disturbance, urinary retention
- Sedation
- Decreased sweating
- Weight gain (may be unusual at low doses)
- Sexual dysfunction
- Metabolic effects, glucose tolerance

 Life Threatening or Dangerous Side Effects
- Rare neuroleptic malignant syndrome
- Rare seizures
- Rare jaundice, agranulocytosis

Weight Gain

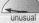
unusual   not unusual   common   problematic

• Reported but not expected especially at low doses

Sedation

unusual not unusual **common** problematic

• Many experience and/or can be significant in amount, especially at high doses
• Sedation is usually dose-dependent and may not be experienced as sedation but as anxiolytic actions on anxiety and aggression at low doses where cyamemazine may function as an atypical antipsychotic (e.g., <300 mg/day; especially 25–100 mg/day)

What To Do About Side Effects

• Wait
• Wait
• Wait
• For motor symptoms, add an anticholinergic agent
• Reduce the dose
• For sedation, give at night
• Switch to an atypical antipsychotic
• Weight loss, exercise programs, and medical management for high BMIs, diabetes, dyslipidemia

Best Augmenting Agents for Side Effects

• Benztropine or trihexyphenidyl for motor side effects
• Benzodiazepines may be helpful for akathisia
• Many side effects cannot be improved with an augmenting agent

DOSING AND USE

Usual Dosage Range

• 50–300 mg at bedtime for treatment of psychosis
• 25–100 mg for anxiety; duration of treatment 4 weeks
• Children (ages 6 and older): 1–4 mg/kg/day
• Injection: 25–100 mg/day

Dosage Forms

• Tablet 25 mg, 100 mg
• Oral solution 40 mg/mL
• Injection 50 mg/5 mL

How to Dose

• Psychosis: usual maintenance dose 50–300 mg at bedtime; maximum dose 600 mg/day divided into 2 or 3 doses; after 2 weeks consider reducing to lowest effective dose
• Anxiety (adults): usual dose 25–100 mg/day; reduce dose if unacceptable sedation; maximum duration of treatment 4 weeks
• Anxiety (children): usual dose 1–4 mg/kg/day

 Dosing Tips

• Has conventional antipsychotic properties at originally recommended high doses (300 to 600 mg/day)
✳ Binding studies, PET studies and clinical observations suggest that cyamemazine may be "atypical" with low motor side effects or prolactin elevations at low doses (below 300 mg/day)
✳ Clinical evidence suggests substantial anxiolytic benefits at 25–100 mg/day in many patients
✳ Clinical evidence suggests low extrapyramidal side effects, little prolactin elevation yet demonstrable anxiolytic, anti-aggression and antidepressant actions at doses below 300 mg/day
• Robust antipsychotic actions on positive symptoms may require dosing above 300 mg/day
• Low doses up to 100 mg/day may be used to augment partial responders to other conventional or atypical antipsychotics, especially for anxiolytic actions

Overdose

• Extrapyramidal symptoms, sedation, hypotension, coma, respiratory depression

Long-Term Use

• Some side effects may be irreversible (e.g., tardive dyskinesia)

Habit Forming

• No

How to Stop

• Slow down titration (over 6 to 8 weeks), especially when simultaneously beginning a new antipsychotic while switching (i.e., cross titration)

- Rapid oral discontinuation of high doses of phenothiazines in psychotic patients may lead to rebound psychosis and worsening of symptoms
- If antiparkinsonian agents are being used, they should generally be continued for a few weeks after high dose cyamemazine is discontinued

Pharmacokinetics

- Half-life 10 hours

 Drug Interactions

- May decrease the effects of levodopa; contraindicated for use with dopamine agonists other than levodopa
- May increase the effects of antihypertensive drugs except for guanethidine, whose antihypertensive actions phenothiazines may antagonize
- May enhance QTc prolongation of other drugs capable of prolonging QTc interval
- Additive effects may occur if used with CNS depressants
- Anticholinergic effects may occur if used with atropine or related compounds
- Some patients taking a neuroleptic and lithium have developed an encephalopathic syndrome similar to neuroleptic malignant syndrome
- Epinephrine may lower blood pressure; diuretics and alcohol may increase risk of hypotension when administered with a phenothiazine

 Other Warnings/ Precautions

- If signs of neuroleptic malignant syndrome develop, treatment should be immediately discontinued
- Use cautiously in patients with respiratory disorders
- Use cautiously in patients with alcohol withdrawal or convulsive disorders because phenothiazines can lower seizure threshold
- Do not use epinephrine in event of overdose as interaction with some pressor agents may lower blood pressure
- Avoid undue exposure to sunlight
- Avoid extreme heat exposure

- Use with caution in patients with respiratory disorders, glaucoma or urinary retention
- Antiemetic effects of phenothiazines may mask signs of other disorders or overdose; suppression of cough reflex may cause asphyxia
- Observe for signs of ocular toxicity (corneal and lenticular deposits) as for other phenothiazines
- Use only with caution or at low doses, if at all, in Parkinson's disease or Lewy Body dementia
- Because cyamemazine may dose-dependently prolong QTc interval, use with caution in patients who have bradycardia or who are taking drugs that can induce bradycardia (e.g., beta blockers, calcium channel blockers, clonidine, digitalis)
- Because cyamemazine may dose-dependently prolong QTc interval, use with caution in patients who have hyperkalemia and/or hypomagnesemia or who are taking drugs that can induce hypokalemia and/or magnesemia (e.g., diuretics, stimulant laxatives, intravenous amphotericin B, glucocorticoids, tetracosaclides)
- Cyamemazine can increase the QTc interval, potentially causing torsades de pointes-type arrhythmia or sudden death

Do Not Use

- If there is a history of QTc prolongation or cardiac arrhythmia, recent acute myocardial infarction, uncompensated heart failure
- ✳ If QTc interval greater than 450 msec or if taking an agent capable of prolonging the QTc interval
- If patient is taking sultopride
- If patient is in a comatose state or has CNS depression
- If there is the presence of blood dyscrasias, bone marrow depression, or liver disease
- If there is subcortical brain damage
- If patient has sensitivity to or intolerance of gluten (tablets contain gluten)
- If patient has congenital galactosemy, does not adequately absorb glucose/galactose, or has lactase deficit (tablets contain lactose)
- If patient is intolerant of fructose, does not adequately absorb glucose/galactose, or

has sugar-isomaltase deficit (oral solution only; oral solution contains saccharose)
- If there is a proven allergy to cyamemazine
- If there is a known sensitivity to any phenothiazine

SPECIAL POPULATIONS

Renal Impairment
- Use with caution

Hepatic Impairment
- Use with caution

Cardiac Impairment
- Cardiovacular toxicity can occur, especially orthostatic hypotension

Elderly
- Elderly patients may be more susceptible to adverse effects
- Lower doses should be used and patient should be monitored closely
- Generally, doses above 100 mg/day are not recommended

Children and Adolescents
- Sometimes used for severe behavioral disturbances in children ages 6 and older
- Oral solution is preferable to the other formulations

Pregnancy
- Phenothiazines are considered risk category C [some animal studies show adverse effects, no controlled studies in humans]
- Reports of extrapyramidal symptoms, jaundice, hyperreflexia, hyporeflexia in infants whose mothers took a phenothiazine during pregnancy
- Phenothiazines should only be used during pregnancy if clearly needed
- Psychotic symptoms may worsen during pregnancy and some form of treatment may be necessary
- Atypical antipsychotics may be preferable to phenothiazines or anticonvulsant mood stabilizers if treatment is required during pregnancy

Breast Feeding
- Unknown if cyamemazine is secreted in human breast milk, but all psychotropics assumed to be secreted in breast milk
- ✳ Recommended either to discontinue drug or bottle feed

THE ART OF PSYCHOPHARMACOLOGY

Potential Advantages
- For anxiety in patients with psychotic illnesses
- For anxiety in patients with non-psychotic illnesses
- For severe depression

Potential Disadvantages
- Patients with tardive dyskinesia
- Children
- Elderly

Primary Target Symptoms
- Anxiety associated with psychosis
- Anxiety
- Aggression
- Agitation
- Positive symptoms of psychosis
- Severe depression

Pearls
- One of the most frequently prescribed antipsychotics in France, especially as a low dose anxiolytic for psychotic patients
- ✳ Appears to have unique anxiolytic actions at low doses without rebound anxiety following discontinuation
- ✳ Low doses rarely associated with motor side effects or with prolactin elevation
- ✳ Recently discovered to be a serotonin dopamine antagonist with more potent binding of 5HT2A and 5HT2C receptors than D2 receptors (binding studies and PET scans)
- Low doses appear to saturate 5HT2A receptors in frontal cortex while not saturating D2 receptors in the striatum, accounting for apparent atypical antipsychotic and anxiolytic properties at low doses
- May be useful second line therapy in facilitating benzodiazepine withdrawal for those patients in whom substitution with

another benzodiazepine is not effective or is not appropriate

Suggested Reading

Lemoine P, Kermadi I, Garcia-Acosta S, Garay RP, Dib M. Double-blind, comparative study of cyamemazine vs. bromazepam in the benzodiazepine withdrawal syndrome. Prog Neuropsychopharmacol Biol Psychiatry 2006;30(1):131–7.

Hameg A, Bayle F, Nuss P, Dupuis P, Garay RP, Dib M. Affinity of cyamemazine, an anxiolytic antipsychotic drug, for human recombinant dopamine vs. serotonin receptor subtypes. Biochem Pharmacol 2003;65(3):435–40.

Hode Y, Reimold M, Demazieres A, Reischl G, Bayle F, Nuss P et al. A positron emission tomography (PET) study of cerebral dopamine D2 and serotonine 5-HT2A receptor occupancy in patients treated with cyamemazine (Tercian). Psychopharmacology (Berl) 2005;180(2):377–84.

GABAPENTIN

THERAPEUTICS

Brands • Neurontin
see index for additional brand names

Generic? Not in U.S. or Europe

 Class

- Anticonvulsant, antineuralgic for chronic pain, alpha 2 delta ligand at voltage-sensitive calcium channels

Commonly Prescribed For
(bold for FDA approved)
- **Partial seizures with or without secondary generalization (adjunctive)**
- **Postherpetic neuralgia**
- Neuropathic pain/chronic pain
- Anxiety (adjunctive)
- Bipolar disorder (adjunctive)

 How The Drug Works

- Is a leucine analogue and is transported both into the blood from the gut and also across the blood-brain barrier into the brain from the blood by the system L transport system
- ✳ Binds to the alpha 2 delta subunit of voltage-sensitive calcium channels
- This closes N and P/Q presynaptic calcium channels, diminishing excessive neuronal activity and neurotransmitter release
- Although structurally related to gamma-aminobutyric acid (GABA), no known direct actions on GABA or its receptors

How Long Until It Works
- Should reduce seizures by 2 weeks
- Should also reduce pain in postherpetic neuralgia by 2 weeks; some patients respond earlier
- May reduce pain in other neuropathic pain syndromes within a few weeks
- If it is not reducing pain within 6–8 weeks, it may require a dosage increase or it may not work at all
- May reduce anxiety in a variety of disorders within a few weeks
- Not yet clear if it has mood stabilizing effects in bipolar disorder or antineuralgic actions in chronic neuropathic pain, but some patients may respond and if so, would be expected to show clinical effects

starting by 2 weeks although it may take several weeks to months to optimize

If It Works
- The goal of treatment is complete remission of symptoms (e.g., seizures)
- The goal of treatment of chronic neuropathic pain is to reduce symptoms as much as possible, especially in combination with other treatments
- Treatment of chronic neuropathic pain most often reduces but does not eliminate symptoms and is not a cure since symptoms usually recur after medicine stopped
- Continue treatment until all symptoms are gone or until improvement is stable and then continue treating indefinitely as long as improvement persists

If It Doesn't Work (for neuropathic pain or bipolar disorder)
- ✳ May only be effective in a subset of bipolar patients, in some patients who fail to respond to other mood stabilizers, or it may not work at all
- Many patients only have a partial response where some symptoms are improved but others persist or continue to wax and wane without stabilization of pain or mood
- Other patients may be nonresponders, sometimes called treatment-resistant or treatment-refractory
- Consider increasing dose, switching to another agent or adding an appropriate augmenting agent
- Consider biofeedback or hypnosis for pain
- Consider the presence of noncompliance and counsel patient
- Switch to another agent with fewer side effects
- Consider evaluation for another diagnosis or for a comorbid condition (e.g., medical illness, substance abuse, etc.)

 Best Augmenting Combos for Partial Response or Treatment-Resistance
- ✳ Gabapentin is itself an augmenting agent to numerous other anticonvulsants in treating epilepsy; and to lithium, atypical antipsychotics and other anticonvulsants in the treatment of bipolar disorder
- For postherpetic neuralgia, gabapentin can decrease concomitant opiate use

✱ For neuropathic pain, gabapentin can augment tricyclic antidepressants and SNRIs as well as tiagabine, other anticonvulsants and even opiates if done by experts while carefully monitoring in difficult cases
• For anxiety, gabapentin is a second-line treatment to augment SSRIs, SNRIs, or benzodiazepines

Tests
• None for healthy individuals
• False positive readings with the Ames N-Multistix SG® dipstick test for urinary protein have been reported when gabapentin was administered with other anticonvulsants

• Dose-related; can be problematic at high doses
• Can wear off with time, but may not wear off at high doses

What To Do About Side Effects
• Wait
• Wait
• Wait
• Take more of the dose at night to reduce daytime sedation
• Lower the dose
• Switch to another agent

Best Augmenting Agents for Side Effects
• Many side effects cannot be improved with an augmenting agent

SIDE EFFECTS

How Drug Causes Side Effects
• CNS side effects may be due to excessive blockade of voltage-sensitive calcium channels

Notable Side Effects
✱ Sedation, dizziness, ataxia, fatigue, nystagmus, tremor
• Vomiting, dyspepsia, diarrhea, dry mouth, constipation, weight gain
• Blurred vision
• Peripheral edema
• Additional effects in children under age 12: hostility, emotional lability, hyperkinesia, thought disorder, weight gain

 Life Threatening or Dangerous Side Effects
• Sudden unexplained deaths have occurred in epilepsy (unknown if related to gabapentin use)

Weight Gain

unusual   not unusual   common   problematic
• Occurs in significant minority

Sedation

unusual   not unusual   common   problematic
• Many experience and/or can be significant in amount

DOSING AND USE

Usual Dosage Range
• 900–1800 mg/day in 3 divided doses

Dosage Forms
• Capsule 100 mg, 300 mg, 400 mg
• Tablet 600 mg, 800 mg
• Liquid 250 mg/5 mL – 470 mL bottle

How to Dose
• Postherpetic neuralgia: 300 mg on day 1; on day 2 increase to 600 mg in 2 doses; on day 3 increase to 900 mg in 3 doses; maximum dose generally 1800 mg/day in 3 doses
• Seizures (ages 12 and older): Initial 900 mg/day in 3 doses; recommended dose generally 1800 mg/day in 3 doses; maximum dose generally 3600 mg/day; time between any 2 doses should usually not exceed 12 hours
• Seizures (under age 13): see Children and Adolescents

 Dosing Tips
• Gabapentin should not be taken until 2 hours after administration of an antacid
• If gabapentin is added to a second anticonvulsant, the titration period should be at least a week to improve tolerance to sedation

- Some patients need to take gabapentin only twice daily in order to experience adequate symptomatic relief for pain or anxiety
- At the high end of the dosing range, tolerability may be enhanced by splitting dose into more than 3 divided doses
- For intolerable sedation, can give most of the dose at night and less during the day
- To improve slow-wave sleep, may only need to take gabapentin at bedtime

Overdose
- No fatalities; slurred speech, sedation, double vision, diarrhea

Long-Term Use
- Safe

Habit Forming
- No

How to Stop
- Taper over a minimum of 1 week
- Epilepsy patients may seize upon withdrawal, especially if withdrawal is abrupt
- ✳ Rapid discontinuation may increase the risk of relapse in bipolar disorder
- Discontinuation symptoms uncommon

Pharmacokinetics
- Gabapentin is not metabolized but excreted intact renally
- Not protein bound
- Elimination half-life approximately 5–7 hours

 Drug Interactions
- Antacids may reduce the bioavailability of gabapentin, so gabapentin should be administered approximately 2 hours before antacid medication
- Naproxen may increase absorption of gabapentin
- Morphine and hydrocodone may increase plasma AUC (area under the curve) values of gabapentin and thus gabapentin plasma levels over time

 Other Warnings/ Precautions
- Depressive effects may be increased by other CNS depressants (alcohol, MAOIs, other anticonvulsants, etc.)
- Dizziness and sedation could increase the chances of accidental injury (falls) in the elderly
- Pancreatic acinar adenocarcinomas have developed in male rats that were given gabapentin, but clinical significance is unknown
- Development of new tumors or worsening of tumors has occurred in humans taking gabapentin; it is unknown whether gabapentin affected the development or worsening of tumors

Do Not Use
- If there is a proven allergy to gabapentin or pregabalin

SPECIAL POPULATIONS

Renal Impairment
- Gabapentin is renally excreted, so the dose may need to be lowered
- Dosing can be adjusted according to creatinine clearance, such that patients with clearance below 16 mL/min should receive 100–300 mg/day in 1 dose, patients with clearance between 16–29 mL/min should receive 200–700 mg/day in 1 dose, and patients with clearance between 30–59 mL/min should receive 400–1400 mg/day in 2 doses
- Can be removed by hemodialysis; patients receiving hemodialysis may require supplemental doses of gabapentin
- Use in renal impairment has not been studied in children under age 12

Hepatic Impairment
- No available data but not metabolized by the liver and clinical experience suggests normal dosing

Cardiac Impairment
- No specific recommendations

Elderly
- Some patients may tolerate lower doses better

- Elderly patients may be more susceptible to adverse effects

Children and Adolescents
- Approved for use starting at age 3 as adjunct treatment for partial seizures
- Ages 5–12: initial 10–15 mg/kg/day in 3 doses; titrate over 3 days to 25–35 mg/kg/day given in 3 doses; maximum dose generally 50 mg/kg/day; time between any 2 doses should usually not exceed 12 hours
- Ages 3–4: initial 10–15 mg/kg/day in 3 doses; titrate over 3 days to 40 mg/kg/day; maximum dose generally 50 mg/kg/day; time between any 2 doses should usually not exceed 12 hours

Pregnancy
- Risk category C [some animal studies show adverse effects, no controlled studies in humans]
- Use in women of childbearing potential requires weighing potential benefits to the mother against the risks to the fetus
- Antiepileptic Drug Pregnancy Registry: (888) 233-2334
- Taper drug if discontinuing
- Seizures, even mild seizures, may cause harm to the embryo/fetus
- ❋ Lack of convincing efficacy for treatment of bipolar disorder or psychosis suggests risk/benefit ratio is in favor of discontinuing gabapentin during pregnancy for these indications
- ❋ For bipolar patients, gabapentin should generally be discontinued before anticipated pregnancies
- ❋ For bipolar patients, given the risk of relapse in the postpartum period, mood stabilizer treatment, especially with agents with better evidence of efficacy than gabapentin, should generally be restarted immediately after delivery if patient is unmedicated during pregnancy
- ❋ Atypical antipsychotics may be preferable to gabapentin if treatment of bipolar disorder is required during pregnancy
- Bipolar symptoms may recur or worsen during pregnancy and some form of treatment may be necessary

Breast Feeding
- Some drug is found in mother's breast milk
- ❋ Recommended either to discontinue drug or bottle feed
- If drug is continued while breast feeding, infant should be monitored for possible adverse effects
- If infant becomes irritable or sedated, breast feeding or drug may need to be discontinued
- ❋ Bipolar disorder may recur during the postpartum period, particularly if there is a history of prior postpartum episodes of either depression or psychosis
- ❋ Relapse rates may be lower in women who receive prophylactic treatment for postpartum episodes of bipolar disorder
- Atypical antipsychotics and anticonvulsants such as valproate may be safer and more effective than gabapentin during the postpartum period when treating a nursing mother with bipolar disorder

---

THE ART OF PSYCHOPHARMACOLOGY

Potential Advantages
- Chronic neuropathic pain
- Has relatively mild side effect profile
- Has few pharmacokinetic drug interactions
- Treatment-resistant bipolar disorder

Potential Disadvantages
- Usually requires 3 times a day dosing
- Poor documentation of efficacy for many off-label uses, especially bipolar disorder

Primary Target Symptoms
- Seizures
- Pain
- Anxiety

Pearls
- Gabapentin is generally well-tolerated, with only mild adverse effects
- Well-studied in epilepsy and postherpetic neuralgia
- ❋ Most use is off-label
- ❋ Off-label use for first-line treatment of neuropathic pain may be justified
- ❋ Off-label use for second-line treatment of anxiety may be justified

✳ Off-label use as an adjunct for bipolar disorder may not be justified
✳ Misperceptions about gabapentin's efficacy in bipolar disorder have led to its use in more patients than other agents with proven efficacy, such as lamotrigine
✳ Off-label use as an adjunct for schizophrenia may not be justified
• May be useful for some patients in alcohol withdrawal

✳ One of the few agents that enhances slow-wave delta sleep, which may be helpful in chronic neuropathic pain syndromes
✳ May be a useful adjunct for fibromyalgia
• Drug absorption and clinical efficacy may not necessarily be proportionately increased at high doses, and thus response to high doses may not be consistent

Suggested Reading

Backonja NM. Use of anticonvulsants for treatment of neuropathic pain. Neurology 2002;59(Suppl 2):S14–7.

MacDonald KJ, Young LT. Newer antiepileptic drugs in bipolar disorder. CNS Drugs 2002;16:549–62.

Marson AG, Kadir ZA, Hutton JL, Chadwick DW. Gabapentin for drug-resistant partial epilepsy. Cochrane Database Syst Rev. 2000;(2):CD001415.

Rose MA, Kam PC. Gabapentin: pharmacology and its use in pain management. Anaesthesia. 2002;57:451–62.

Stahl SM. Anticonvulsants and the relief of chronic pain: pregabalin and gabapentin as alpha(2)delta ligands at voltage-gated calcium channels. J Clin Psychiatry. 2004;65:596–7.

Stahl SM. Anticonvulsants as anxiolytics, part 2: Pregabalin and gabapentin as alpha(2)delta ligands at voltage-gated calcium channels. J Clin Psychiatry. 2004;65:460–1.

LAMOTRIGINE

THERAPEUTICS

Brands
- Lamictal
- Labileno
- Lamictin

see index for additional brand names

Generic? No

Class
- Anticonvulsant, mood stabilizer, voltage-sensitive sodium channel antagonist

Commonly Prescribed For
(bold for FDA approved)
- **Maintenance treatment of bipolar I disorder**
- **Partial seizures (adjunctive; adults and children over age 2)**
- **Generalized seizures of Lennox-Gastaut syndrome (adjunctive; adults and children over age 2)**
- **Conversion to monotherapy in adults with partial seizures who are receiving treatment with carbamazepine, phenytoin, phenobarbital, primidone, or valproate**
- Bipolar depression
- Bipolar mania (adjunctive and second-line)
- Psychosis, schizophrenia (adjunctive)
- Neuropathic pain/chronic pain
- Major depressive disorder (adjunctive)
- Other seizure types and as initial monotherapy for epilepsy

How The Drug Works
* Acts as a use-dependent blocker of voltage-sensitive sodium channels
* Interacts with the open channel conformation of voltage-sensitive sodium channels
* Interacts at a specific site of the alpha pore-forming subunit of voltage-sensitive sodium channels
- Inhibits release of glutamate and asparate

How Long Until It Works
- May take several weeks to improve bipolar depression
- May take several weeks to months to optimize an effect on mood stabilization
- Can reduce seizures by 2 weeks, but may take several weeks to months to reduce seizures

If It Works
- The goal of treatment is complete remission of symptoms (e.g., seizures, depression, pain)
- Continue treatment until all symptoms are gone or until improvement is stable and then continue treating indefinitely as long as improvement persists
- Continue treatment indefinitely to avoid recurrence of mania, depression, and/or seizures
- Treatment of chronic neuropathic pain may reduce but does not eliminate pain symptoms and is not a cure since pain usually recurs after medicine stopped

If It Doesn't Work (for bipolar disorder)
* Many patients only have a partial response where some symptoms are improved but others persist or continue to wax and wane without stabilization of mood
- Other patients may be nonresponders, sometimes called treatment-resistant or treatment-refractory
- Consider increasing dose, switching to another agent or adding an appropriate augmenting agent
- Consider adding psychotherapy
- Consider biofeedback or hypnosis for pain
- Consider the presence of noncompliance and counsel patient
- Switch to another mood stabilizer with fewer side effects
- Consider evaluation for another diagnosis or for a comorbid condition (e.g., medical illness, substance abuse, etc.)

 Best Augmenting Combos for Partial Response or Treatment-Resistance (for bipolar disorder)
- Lithium
- Atypical antipsychotics (especially risperidone, olanzapine, quetiapine, ziprasidone, and aripiprazole)
* Valproate (with caution and at half dose of lamotrigine in the presence of valproate,

because valproate can double lamotrigine levels)

✳ Antidepressants (with caution because antidepressants can destabilize mood in some patients, including induction of rapid cycling or suicidal ideation; in particular consider bupropion; also SSRIs, SNRIs, others; generally avoid TCAs, MAOIs)

Tests
• None required
• The value of monitoring plasma concentrations of lamotrigine has not been established
• Because lamotrigine binds to melanin-containing tissues, opthalmological checks may be considered

SIDE EFFECTS

How Drug Causes Side Effects
• CNS side effects theoretically due to excessive actions at voltage-sensitive sodium channels
• Rash hypothetically an allergic reaction

Notable Side Effects
✳ Benign rash (approximately 10%)
• Sedation, blurred or double vision, dizziness, ataxia, headache, tremor, insomnia, poor coordination, fatigue
• Nausea, vomiting, dyspepsia, abdominal pain, constipation, rhinitis
• Additional effects in pediatric patients with epilepsy: infection, pharyngitis, asthenia

 Life Threatening or Dangerous Side Effects

✳ Rare serious rash (risk may be greater in pediatric patients but still rare)
• Rare multi-organ failure associated with Stevens Johnson syndrome, toxic epidermal necrolysis or drug hypersensitivity syndrome
• Rare blood dyscrasias
• Rare sudden unexplained deaths have occurred in epilepsy (unknown if related to lamotrigine use)
• Withdrawal seizures upon abrupt withdrawal

Weight Gain

unusual   not unusual   common   problematic
• Reported but not expected

Sedation

unusual   not unusual   common   problematic
• Reported but not expected
• Dose-related
• Can wear off with time

What To Do About Side Effects
• Wait
• Take at night to reduce daytime sedation
• Divide dosing to twice daily
✳ If patient develops signs of a rash with benign characteristics (i.e., a rash that peaks within days, settles in 10–14 days, is spotty, nonconfluent, nontender, has no systemic features, and laboratory tests are normal):
  • Reduce lamotrigine dose or stop dosage increase
  • Warn patient to stop drug and contact physician if rash worsens or new symptoms emerge
  • Prescribe antihistamine and/or topical corticosteroid for pruritis
  • Monitor patient closely
✳ If patient develops signs of a rash with serious characteristics (i.e., a rash that is confluent and widespread, or purpuric or tender; with any prominent involvement of neck or upper trunk; any involvement of eyes, lips, mouth, etc.; any associated fever, malaise, pharyngitis, anorexia, or lymphadenopathy; abnormal laboratory tests for complete blood count, liver function, urea, creatinine):
  • Stop lamotrigine (and valproate if administered)
  • Monitor and investigate organ involvement (hepatic, renal, hematologic)
  • Patient may require hospitalization
  • Monitor patient very closely

Best Augmenting Agents for Side Effects
• Antihistamines and/or topical corticosteroid for rash, pruritis
• Many side effects cannot be improved with an augmenting agent

DOSING AND USE

Usual Dosage Range
- Monotherapy for bipolar disorder: 100–200 mg/day
- Adjunctive treatment for bipolar disorder: 100 mg/day in combination with valproate; 400 mg/day in combination with enzyme-inducing antiepileptic drugs such as carbamazepine, phenobarbital, phenytoin, and primidone
- Monotherapy for seizures in patients over age 12: 300–500 mg/day in 2 doses
- Adjunctive treatment for seizures in patients over age 12: 100–400 mg/day for regimens containing valproate; 100–200 mg/day for valproate alone; 300–500 mg/day in 2 doses for regimens not containing valproate
- Patients ages 2–12 with epilepsy are dosed based on body weight and concomitant medications

Dosage Forms
- Tablet 25 mg scored, 100 mg scored, 150 mg scored, 200 mg scored
- Chewable tablet 2 mg, 5 mg, 25 mg

How to Dose
✳ Bipolar disorder (monotherapy): for the first 2 weeks administer 25 mg/day; at week 3 increase to 50 mg/day; at week 5 increase to 100 mg/day; at week 6 increase to 200 mg/day; maximum dose generally 200 mg/day
✳ Bipolar disorder (adjunct to valproate): for the first 2 weeks administer 25 mg every other day; at week 3 increase to 25 mg/day; at week 5 increase to 50 mg/day; at week 6 increase to 100 mg/day; maximum dose generally 100 mg/day
- Bipolar disorder (adjunct to enzyme-inducing antiepileptic drugs): for the first 2 weeks administer 50 mg/day; at week 3 increase to 100 mg/day in divided doses; starting at week 5 increase by 100 mg/day each week; maximum dose generally 400 mg/day in divided doses
- When lamotrigine is added to epilepsy treatment that includes valproate (ages 12 and older): for the first 2 weeks administer 25 mg every other day; at week 3 increase to 25 mg/day; every 1–2 weeks can increase by 25–50 mg/day; usual maintenance dose 100–400 mg/day in 1–2 doses or 100–200 mg/day if lamotrigine is added to valproate alone
- When lamotrigine is added to epilepsy treatment that includes carbamazepine, phenytoin, phenobarbital, or primidone (without valproate) (ages 12 and older): for the first 2 weeks administer 50 mg/day; at week 3 increase to 100 mg/day in 2 doses; every 1–2 weeks can increase by 100 mg/day; usual maintenance dose 300–500 mg/day in 2 doses
- When converting from a single enzyme-inducing antiepileptic drug to lamotrigine monotherapy for epilepsy: titrate as described above to 500 mg/day in 2 doses while maintaining dose of previous medication; decrease first drug in 20% decrements each week over the next 4 weeks
- When converting from valproate to lamotrigine monotherapy for epilepsy: titrate as described above to 200 mg/day while maintaining dose of valproate, then gradually increase lamotrigine up to 500 mg/day while gradually discontinuing valproate
- Seizures (under age 12): see Children and Adolescents

 Dosing Tips
✳ Very slow dose titration may reduce the incidence of skin rash
- Therefore, dose should not be titrated faster than recommended because of possible risk of increased side effects, including rash
- If patient stops taking lamotrigine for 5 days or more it may be necessary to restart the drug with the initial dose titration, as rashes have been reported on re-exposure
- Advise patient to avoid new medications, foods, or products during the first 3 months of lamotrigine treatment in order to decrease the risk of unrelated rash; patient should also not start lamotrigine within 2 weeks of a viral infection, rash, or vaccination
✳ If lamotrigine is added to patients taking valproate, remember that valproate inhibits lamotrigine metabolism and therefore titration rate and ultimate dose of

lamotrigine should be reduced by 50% to reduce the risk of rash

✳ Thus, if concomitant valproate is discontinued after lamotrigine dose is stabilized, then the lamotrigine dose should be cautiously doubled over at least 2 weeks in equal increments each week following discontinuation of valproate

• Also, if concomitant enzyme-inducing antiepileptic drugs such as carbamazepine, phenobarbital, phenytoin, and primidone are discontinued after lamotrigine dose is stabilized, then the lamotrigine dose should be maintained for 1 week following discontinuation of the other drug and then reduced by half over 2 weeks in equal decrements each week

• Since oral contraceptives and pregnancy can decrease lamotrigine levels, adjustments to the maintenance dose of lamotrigine are recommended in women taking, starting, or stopping oral contraceptives, becoming pregnant, or after delivery

• Chewable dispersible tablets should only be administered as whole tablets; dose should be rounded down to the nearest whole tablet

• Chewable dispersible tablets can be dispersed by adding the tablet to liquid (enough to cover the drug); after approximately 1 minute the solution should be stirred and then consumed immediately in its entirety

Overdose

• Some fatalities have occurred; ataxia, nystagmus, seizures, coma, intraventricular conduction delay

Long-Term Use

• Safe

Habit Forming

• No

How to Stop

• Taper over at least 2 weeks
✳ Rapid discontinuation can increase the risk of relapse in bipolar disorder
• Patients with epilepsy may seize upon withdrawal, especially if withdrawal is abrupt
• Discontinuation symptoms uncommon

Pharmacokinetics

• Elimination half-life in healthy volunteers approximately 33 hours after a single dose of lamotrigine

• Elimination half-life in patients receiving concomitant valproate treatment approximately 59 hours after a single dose of lamotrigine

• Elimination half-life in patients receiving concomitant enzyme-inducing antiepileptic drugs (such as carbamazepine, phenobarbital, phenytoin, and primidone) approximately 14 hours after a single dose of lamotrigine

• Metabolized in the liver through glucorunidation but not through the CYP450 enzyme system

• Inactive metabolite

• Renally excreted

• Lamotrigine inhibits dihydrofolate reductase and may therefore reduce folate concentrations

• Rapidly and completely absorbed; bioavailability not affected by food

 Drug Interactions

✳ Valproate increases plasma concentrations and half-life of lamotrigine, requiring lower doses of lamotrigine (half or less)

✳ Use of lamotrigine with valproate may be associated with an increased incidence of rash

• Enzyme-inducing antiepileptic drugs (e.g., carbamazepine, phenobarbital, phenytoin, primidone) may increase the clearance of lamotrigine and lower its plasma levels

• Oral contraceptives may decrease plasma levels of lamotrigine

• No likely pharmacokinetic interactions of lamotrigine with lithium, oxcarbazepine, atypical antipsychotics, or antidepressants

 Other Warnings/ Precautions

✳ Life-threatening rashes have developed in association with lamotrigine use; lamotrigine should generally be discontinued at the first sign of serious rash

✳ Risk of rash may be increased with higher doses, faster dose escalation,

concomitant use of valproate, or in children under age 12
- Patient should be instructed to report any symptoms of hypersensitivity immediately (fever; flu-like symptoms; rash; blisters on skin or in eyes, mouth, ears, nose, or genital areas; swelling of eyelids, conjunctivitis, lymphadenopathy)
- Depressive effects may be increased by other CNS depressants (alcohol, MAOIs, other anticonvulsants, etc.)
- A small number of people may experience a worsening of seizures
- May cause photosensitivity
- Lamotrigine binds to tissue that contains melanin, so for long-term treatment ophthalmological checks may be considered

Do Not Use
- If there is a proven allergy to lamotrigine

SPECIAL POPULATIONS

Renal Impairment
- Lamotrigine is renally excreted, so the maintenance dose may need to be lowered
- Can be removed by hemodialysis; patients receiving hemodialysis may require supplemental doses of lamotrigine

Hepatic Impairment
- Dose may need to be reduced and titration may need to be slower, perhaps by 50% in patients with moderate impairment and 75% in patients with severe impairment

Cardiac Impairment
- Clinical experience is limited
- Drug should be used with caution

Elderly
- Some patients may tolerate lower doses better
- Elderly patients may be more susceptible to adverse effects

 Children and Adolescents
- Ages 2 and older: approved as add-on for Lennox-Gastaut syndrome
- Ages 2 and older: approved as add-on for partial seizures

- No other use of lamotrigine is approved for patients under 16 years of age
- ✳ Risk of rash is increased in pediatric patients, especially in children under 12 and in children taking valproate
- When lamotrigine is added to treatment that includes valproate (ages 2–12): for the first 2 weeks administer 0.15 mg/kg/day in 1–2 doses rounded down to the nearest whole tablet; at week 3 increase to 0.3 mg/kg/day in 1–2 doses rounded down to the nearest whole tablet; every 1–2 weeks can increase by 0.3 mg/kg/day rounded down to the nearest whole tablet; usual maintenance dose 1–5 mg/kg/day in 1–2 doses (maximum generally 200 mg/day) or 1–3 mg/kg/day in 1–2 doses if lamotrigine is added to valproate alone
- When lamotrigine is added to treatment with carbamazepine, phenytoin, phenobarbital, or primidone (without valproate) (ages 2–12): for the first 2 weeks administer 0.6 mg/kg/day in 2 doses rounded down to the nearest whole tablet; at week 3 increase to 1.2 mg/kg/day in 2 doses rounded down to the nearest whole tablet; every 1–2 weeks can increase by 1.2 mg/kg/day rounded down to the nearest whole tablet; usual maintenance dose 5–15 mg/kg/day in 2 doses (maximum dose generally 400 mg/day)
- Clearance of lamotrigine may be influenced by weight, such that patients weighing less than 30 kg may require an increase of up to 50% for maintenance doses

 Pregnancy
- Risk category C [some animal studies show adverse effects, no controlled studies in humans]
- Use in women of childbearing potential requires weighing potential benefits to the mother against the risks to the fetus
- ✳ If treatment with lamotrigine is continued, plasma concentrations of lamotrigine may be reduced during pregnancy, possibly requiring increased doses with dose reduction following delivery
- Pregnancy exposure registry for lamotrigine: (800) 336-2176
- Taper drug if discontinuing

- Seizures, even mild seizures, may cause harm to the embryo/fetus
- Recurrent bipolar illness during pregnancy can be quite disruptive
* For bipolar patients, lamotrigine should generally be discontinued before anticipated pregnancies
* For bipolar patients in whom treatment is discontinued, given the risk of relapse in the postpartum period, lamotrigine should generally be restarted immediately after delivery
* Atypical antipsychotics may be preferable to lithium or anticonvulsants such as lamotrigine if treatment of bipolar disorder is required during pregnancy, but lamotrigine may be preferable to other anticonvulsants such as valproate if anticonvulsant treatment is required during pregnancy
- Bipolar symptoms may recur or worsen during pregnancy and some form of treatment may be necessary

Breast Feeding
- Some drug is found in mother's breast milk
* Generally recommended either to discontinue drug or bottle feed
- If drug is continued while breast feeding, infant should be monitored for possible adverse effects
- If infant shows signs of irritability or sedation, drug may need to be discontinued
* Bipolar disorder may recur during the postpartum period, particularly if there is a history of prior postpartum episodes of either depression or psychosis
* Relapse rates may be lower in women who receive prophylactic treatment for postpartum episodes of bipolar disorder
- Atypical antipsychotics and anticonvulsants such as valproate may be preferable to lithium or lamotrigine during the postpartum period when breast feeding

THE ART OF PSYCHOPHARMACOLOGY

Potential Advantages
- Depressive stages of bipolar disorder (bipolar depression)
- To prevent recurrences of both depression and mania in bipolar disorder

Potential Disadvantages
- May not be as effective in the manic stage of bipolar disorder

Primary Target Symptoms
- Incidence of seizures
- Unstable mood, especially depression, in bipolar disorder
- Pain

Pearls
* Lamotrigine is a first-line treatment option that may be best for patients with bipolar depression
* Seems to be more effective in treating depressive episodes than manic episodes in bipolar disorder (treats from below better than it treats from above)
* Seems to be effective in preventing both manic relapses as well as depressive relapses (stabilizes both from above and from below) although it may be even better for preventing depressive relapses than for preventing manic relapses
* Despite convincing evidence of efficacy in bipolar disorder, is often used less frequently than anticonvulsants without convincing evidence of efficacy in bipolar disorder (e.g., gabapentin or topiramate)
* Low levels of use may be based upon exaggerated fears of skin rashes or lack of knowledge about how to manage skin rashes if they occur
* May actually be one of the best tolerated mood stabilizers with little weight gain or sedation
- Actual risk of serious skin rash may be comparable to agents erroneously considered "safer" including carbamazepine, phenytoin, phenobarbital, and zonisamide
- Rashes are common even in placebo-treated patients in clinical trials of bipolar patients (5–10%) due to non-drug related causes including eczema, irritant, and allergic contact dermatitis, such as poison ivy and insect bite reactions
* To manage rashes in bipolar patients receiving lamotrigine, realize that rashes that occur within the first 5 days or after 8–12 weeks of treatment are rarely drug-related, and learn the clinical distinctions

between a benign rash and a serious rash (see What to Do About Side Effects above)
- Rash, including serious rash, appears riskiest in younger children, in those who are receiving concomitant valproate, and/or in those receiving rapid lamotrigine titration and/or high dosing
- Risk of serious rash is less than 1% and has been declining since slower titration, lower dosing, adjustments to use of concomitant valproate administration, and limitations on use in children under 12 have been implemented
- Incidence of serious rash is very low (approaching zero) in recent studies of bipolar patients
- Benign rashes related to lamotrigine may affect up to 10% of patients and resolve rapidly with drug discontinuation
- ❋ Given the limited treatment options for bipolar depression, patients with benign rashes can even be re-challenged with lamotrigine 5–12 mg/day with very slow titration after risk-benefit analysis if they are informed, reliable, closely monitored, and warned to stop lamotrigine and contact their physician if signs of hypersensitivity occur
- Only a third of bipolar patients experience adequate relief with a monotherapy, so most patients need multiple medications for best control
- Lamotrigine is useful in combination with atypical antipsychotics and/or lithium for acute mania
- Usefulness for bipolar disorder in combination with anticonvulsants other than valproate is not well demonstrated; such combinations can be expensive and are possibly ineffective or even irrational
- May be useful as an adjunct to atypical antipsychotics for rapid onset of action in schizophrenia
- May be useful as an adjunct to antidepressants in major depressive disorder
- Early studies suggest possible utility for patients with neuropathic pain such as diabetic peripheral neuropathy, HIV-associated neuropathy, and other pain conditions including migraine

Suggested Reading

Calabrese JR, Bowden CL, Sachs GS et al. A double-blind placebo-controlled study of lamotrigine monotherapy in outpatients with bipolar I depression. J Clin Psych 1999;60:79–88.

Calabrese JR, Sullivan JR, Bowden CL, Suppes T, Goldberg JF, Sachs GS, Shelton MD, Goodwin FK, Frye MA, Kusumakar V. Rash in multicenter trials of lamotrigine in mood disorders: clinical relevance and management. J Clin Psychiatry. 2002;63:1012–1019

Culy CR, Goa KL. Lamotrigine. A review of its use in childhood epilepsy. Paediatr Drugs. 2000; 2: 299–330.

Cunningham M, Tennis P, and the International Lamotrigine Pregnancy Registry Scientific Advisory Committee. Lamotrigine and the risk of malformations in pregnancy. Neurology 2005;64:955–960.

Green B. Lamotrigine in mood disorders. Curr Med Res Opin. 2003;19:272–7.

Goodwin GM, Bowden CL, Calabrese JR et al. A pooled analysis of 2 placebo-controlled 18-month trials of lamotrigine and lithium maintenance treatment in bipolar I disorder. J Clin Psychiatry 2004;65:432–441.

THERAPEUTICS

Brands • Keppra
see index for additional brand names

Generic? No

Class

- Anticonvulsant, synaptic vesicle protein SV2A modulator

Commonly Prescribed For
(bold for FDA approved)

- **Adjunct therapy for partial seizures in adults with epilepsy**
- Neuropathic pain/chronic pain
- Mania

How The Drug Works

- ✳ Binds to synaptic vesicle protein SV2A, which is involved in synaptic vesicle exocytosis
- Opposes the activity of negative modulators of GABA- and glycine-gated currents and partially inhibits N-type calcium currents in neuronal cells

How Long Until It Works

- Should reduce seizures by 2 weeks
- Not yet clear if it has mood stabilizing effects in bipolar disorder or antineuralgic actions in chronic neuropathic pain, but some patients may respond and if so, would be expected to show clinical effects starting by 2 weeks although it may take several weeks to months to optimize clinical effects

If It Works

- The goal of treatment is complete remission of symptoms (e.g., seizures, mania, pain)
- The goal of treatment of chronic neuropathic pain is to reduce symptoms as much as possible, especially in combination with other treatments
- Treatment of chronic neuropathic pain most often reduces but does not eliminate symptoms and is not a cure since symptoms usually recur after medicine stopped
- Continue treatment until all symptoms are gone or until mood is stable and then continue treating indefinitely as long as improvement persists
- Continue treatment indefinitely to avoid recurrence of seizures, mania, and pain

If It Doesn't Work (for bipolar disorder or neuropathic pain)

- ✳ May only be effective in a subset of bipolar patients, in some patients who fail to respond to other mood stabilizers, or it may not work at all
- Many patients only have a partial response where some symptoms are improved but others persist or continue to wax and wane without stabilization of pain or mood
- Other patients may be nonresponders, sometimes called treatment-resistant or treatment-refractory
- Consider increasing dose or switching to another agent with better demonstrated efficacy in bipolar disorder or neuropathic pain

Best Augmenting Combos for Partial Response or Treatment-Resistance

- Levetiracetam is itself a second-line augmenting agent to numerous other anticonvulsants, lithium, and atypical antipsychotics for bipolar disorder and to gabapentin, tiagabine, other anticonvulsants, SNRIs, and tricyclic antidepressants for neuropathic pain

Tests

- None for healthy individuals

SIDE EFFECTS

How Drug Causes Side Effects

- CNS side effects may be due to excessive actions on SV2A synaptic vesicle proteins or to actions on various voltage-sensitive ion channels

Notable Side Effects

- ✳ Sedation, dizziness, ataxia, asthenia
- Hematologic abnormalities (decrease in red blood cell count and hemoglobin)

Life Threatening or Dangerous Side Effects
- Activation of suicidal ideation and acts (rare)

Weight Gain

| unusual | not unusual | common | problematic |

- Reported but not expected

Sedation

| unusual | not unusual | common | problematic |

- Many experience and/or can be significant in amount

What To Do About Side Effects
- Wait
- Wait
- Wait
- Take more of the dose at night to reduce daytime sedation
- Lower the dose
- Switch to another agent

Best Augmenting Agents for Side Effects
- Many side effects cannot be improved with an augmenting agent

DOSING AND USE

Usual Dosage Range
- 1000–3000 mg/day in 2 doses

Dosage Forms
- Tablet 250 mg, 500 mg, 750 mg
- Oral solution 100 mg/mL

How to Dose
- Initial 1000 mg/day in 2 divided doses; after 2 weeks can increase by 1000 mg/day every 2 weeks; maximum dose generally 3000 mg/day

 Dosing Tips
- For intolerable sedation, can give most of the dose at night and less during the day
- Some patients may tolerate and respond to doses greater than 3000 mg/day

Overdose
- No fatalities; sedation, agitation, aggression, respiratory depression, coma

Long-Term Use
- Safe

Habit Forming
- No

How to Stop
- Taper
- Epilepsy patients may seize upon withdrawal, especially if withdrawal is abrupt
- * Rapid discontinuation can increase the risk of relapse in bipolar disorder
- Discontinuation symptoms uncommon

Pharmacokinetics
- Elimination half-life approximately 6–8 hours
- Inactive metabolites
- Not metabolized by CYP450 enzymes
- Does not inhibit/induce CYP450 enzymes
- Renally excreted

 Drug Interactions
- Because levetiracetam is not metabolized by CYP450 enzymes and does not inhibit or induce CYP450 enzymes, it is unlikely to have significant pharmacokinetic drug interactions

 Other Warnings/ Precautions
- Depressive effects may be increased by other CNS depressants (alcohol, MAOIs, other anticonvulsants, etc.)

Do Not Use
- If there is a proven allergy to levetiracetam

SPECIAL POPULATIONS

Renal Impairment
- Recommended dose for patients with mild impairment may be between 500 mg and 1500 mg twice a day
- Recommended dose for patients with moderate impairment may be between 250 mg and 750 mg twice a day

- Recommended dose for patients with severe impairment may be between 250 mg and 500 mg twice a day
- Patients on dialysis may require doses between 500 mg and 1000 mg once a day, with a supplemental dose of 250–500 mg following dialysis

Hepatic Impairment
- Dose adjustment usually not necessary

Cardiac Impairment
- No specific recommendations

Elderly
- Some patients may tolerate lower doses better
- Elderly patients may be more susceptible to adverse effects

 Children and Adolescents
- Safety and efficacy not established under age 16
- Children may require higher doses than adults; dosing should be adjusted according to weight

 Pregnancy
- Risk category C [some animal studies show adverse effects, no controlled studies in humans]
- Use in women of childbearing potential requires weighing potential benefits to the mother against the risks to the fetus
- Antiepileptic Drug Pregnancy Registry: (888) 233-2334
- Taper drug if discontinuing
- Seizures, even mild seizures, may cause harm to the embryo/fetus
- Lack of convincing efficacy for treatment of bipolar disorder or chronic neuropathic pain suggests risk/benefit ratio is in favor of discontinuing levetiracetam during pregnancy for these indications
- ❋ For bipolar patients, given the risk of relapse in the postpartum period, mood stabilizer treatment, especially with agents with better evidence of efficacy than levetiracetam, should generally be restarted immediately after delivery if patient is unmedicated during pregnancy

- ❋ For bipolar patients, levetiracetam should generally be discontinued before anticipated pregnancies
- ❋ Atypical antipsychotics may be preferable to levetiracetam if treatment of bipolar disorder is required during pregnancy
- Bipolar symptoms may recur or worsen during pregnancy and some form of treatment may be necessary

Breast Feeding
- Some drug is found in mother's breast milk
- ❋ Recommended either to discontinue drug or bottle feed
- If drug is continued while breast feeding, infant should be monitored for possible adverse effects
- If infant becomes irritable or sedated, breast feeding or drug may need to be discontinued
- ❋ Bipolar disorder may recur during the postpartum period, particularly if there is a history of prior postpartum episodes of either depression or psychosis
- ❋ Relapse rates may be lower in women who receive prophylactic treatment for postpartum episodes of bipolar disorder
- Atypical antipsychotics and anticonvulsants such as valproate may be safer than levetiracetam during the postpartum period when breast feeding

THE ART OF PSYCHOPHARMACOLOGY

Potential Advantages
- Patients on concomitant drugs (lack of drug interactions)
- Treatment-refractory bipolar disorder
- Treatment-refractory neuropathic pain

Potential Disadvantages
- Patients noncompliant with twice daily dosing
- Efficacy for bipolar disorder or neuropathic pain not well documented

Primary Target Symptoms
- Seizures
- Pain
- Mania

Pearls

- Well studied in epilepsy
- ✳ Off-label use second-line and as an augmenting agent may be justified for bipolar disorder and neuropathic pain unresponsive to other treatments
- ✳ Unique mechanism of action suggests utility where other anticonvulsants fail to work

✳ Unique mechanism of action as modulator of synaptic vesicle release suggests theoretical utility for clinical conditions that are hypothetically linked to excessively activated neuronal circuits, such as anxiety disorders and neuropathic pain as well as epilepsy

Suggested Reading

Ben-Menachem E. Levetiracetam: treatment in epilepsy. Expert Opin Pharmacother. 2003;4(11):2079–88.

French J. Use of levetiracetam in special populations. Epilepsia. 2001;42 Suppl 4:40–3.

Leppik IE. Three new drugs for epilepsy: levetiracetam, oxcarbazepine, and zonisamide. J Child Neurol. 2002;17 Suppl 1:S53–7.

Lynch BA, Lambeng N, Nocka K, Kensel-Hammes P, Bajjalieh SM, Matagne A, Fuks B.. The synaptic vesicle protein SV2A is the binding site for the antiepileptic drug levetiracetam. Proc Natl Acad Sci U S A. 2004;101:9861–6.

Pinto A, Sander JW. Levetiracetam: a new therapeutic option for refractory epilepsy. Int J Clin Pract. 2003;57(7):616–21.

LITHIUM

Brands
- Eskalith
- Eskalith CR
- Lithobid slow release tablets
- Lithostat tablets
- Lithium carbonate tablets
- Lithium citrate syrup

see index for additional brand names

Generic? Yes

Class
- Mood stabilizer

Commonly Prescribed For
(bold for FDA approved)
- **Manic episodes of manic depressive illness**
- **Maintenance treatment for manic depressive patients with a history of mania**
- Bipolar depression
- Major depressive disorder (adjunctive)
- Vascular headache
- Neutropenia

How The Drug Works
- Unknown and complex
- Alters sodium transport across cell membranes in nerve and muscle cells
- Alters metabolism of neurotransmitters including catecholamines and serotonin
- ✳ May alter intracellular signaling through actions on second messenger systems
- Specifically, inhibits inositol monophosphatase, possibly affecting neurotransmission via phosphatidyl inositol second messenger system
- Also reduces protein kinase C activity, possibly affecting genomic expression associated with neurotransmission
- Increases cytoprotective proteins, activates signaling cascade utilized by endogenous growth factors, and increases gray matter content, possibly by activating neurogenesis and enhancing trophic actions that maintain synapses

How Long Until It Works
- 1–3 weeks

If It Works
- The goal of treatment is complete remission of symptoms (i.e., mania and/or depression)
- Continue treatment until all symptoms are gone or until improvement is stable and then continue treating indefinitely as long as improvement persists
- Continue treatment indefinitely to avoid recurrence of mania or depression

If It Doesn't Work
- ✳ Many patients only have a partial response where some symptoms are improved but others persist or continue to wax and wane without stabilization of mood
- Other patients may be nonresponders, sometimes called treatment-resistant or treatment-refractory
- Consider checking plasma drug level, increasing dose, switching to another agent or adding an appropriate augmenting agent
- Consider adding psychotherapy
- Consider the presence of noncompliance and counsel patient
- Switch to another mood stabilizer with fewer side effects
- Consider evaluation for another diagnosis or for a comorbid condition (e.g., medical illness, substance abuse, etc.)

Best Augmenting Combos for Partial Response or Treatment-Resistance
- Valproate
- Atypical antipsychotics (especially risperidone, olanzapine, quetiapine, ziprasidone, and aripiprazole)
- Lamotrigine
- ✳ Antidepressants (with caution because antidepressants can destabilize mood in some patients, including induction of rapid cycling or suicidal ideation; in particular consider bupropion; also SSRIs, SNRIs, others; generally avoid TCAs, MAOIs)

Tests
- ✳ Before initiating treatment, kidney function tests (including creatinine and urine specific gravity) and thyroid function tests; electrocardiogram for patients over 50
- Repeat kidney function tests 1–2 times/year

※ Frequent tests to monitor trough lithium plasma levels (should generally be between 1.0 and 1.5 mEq/L for acute treatment, 0.6 and 1.2 mEq/l for chronic treatment)

※ Since lithium is frequently associated with weight gain, before starting treatment, weigh all patients and determine if the patient is already overweight (BMI 25.0–29.9) or obese (BMI ≥30)

• Before giving a drug that can cause weight gain to an overweight or obese patient, consider determining whether the patient already has pre-diabetes (fasting plasma glucose 100–125 mg/dl), diabetes (fasting plasma glucose >126 mg/dl), or dyslipidemia (increased total cholesterol, LDL cholesterol and triglycerides; decreased HDL cholesterol), and treat or refer such patients for treatment, including nutrition and weight management, physical activity counseling, smoking cessation, and medical management

※ Monitor weight and BMI during treatment

※ While giving a drug to a patient who has gained >5% of initial weight, consider evaluating for the presence of pre-diabetes, diabetes, or dyslipidemia, or consider switching to a different agent

SIDE EFFECTS

How Drug Causes Side Effects
• Unknown and complex
• CNS side effects theoretically due to excessive actions at the same or similar sites that mediate its therapeutic actions
• Some renal side effects theoretically due to lithium's actions on ion transport

Notable Side Effects
※ Ataxia, dysarthria, delirium, tremor, memory problems
※ Polyuria, polydipsia (nephrogenic diabetes insipidus)
※ Diarrhea, nausea
※ Weight gain
• Euthyroid goiter or hypothyroid goiter, possibly with increased TSH and reduced thyroxine levels
• Acne, rash, alopecia
• Leukocytosis
• Side effects are typically dose-related

 Life Threatening or Dangerous Side Effects
• Lithium toxicity
• Renal impairment (interstitial nephritis)
• Nephrogenic diabetes insipidus
• Arrhythmia, cardiovascular changes, sick sinus syndrome, bradycardia, hypotension
• T wave flattening and inversion
• Rare pseudotumor cerebri
• Rare seizures

Weight Gain

unusual   not unusual   common   problematic

• Many experience and/or can be significant in amount
• Can become a health problem in some
• May be associated with increased appetite

Sedation

unusual   not unusual   common   problematic

• Many experience and/or can be significant in amount
• May wear off with time

What To Do About Side Effects
• Wait
• Wait
• Wait
• Lower the dose
※ Take entire dose at night as long as efficacy persists all day long with this administration
※ Change to a different lithium preparation (e.g., controlled release)
※ Reduce dosing from 3 times/day to 2 times/day
• If signs of lithium toxicity occur, discontinue immediately
• For stomach upset, take with food
• For tremor, avoid caffeine
• Switch to another agent

Best Augmenting Agents for Side Effects
※ Propranolol 20–30 mg 2–3 times/day may reduce tremor
• For the expert, cautious addition of a diuretic (e.g., chlorothiazide 50 mg/day) while reducing lithium dose by 50% and monitoring plasma lithium levels may

reduce polydipsia and polyuria that does not go away with time alone
• Many side effects cannot be improved with an augmenting agent

DOSING AND USE

Usual Dosage Range
• 1800 mg/day in divided doses (acute)
• 900–1200 mg/day in divided doses (maintenance)
• Liquid: 10 mL three times/day (acute mania); 5 mL 3–4 times/day (long-term)

Dosage Forms
• Tablet 300 mg (slow release), 450 mg (controlled release)
• Capsule 150 mg, 300 mg, 600 mg
• Liquid 8 mEq/5 mL

How to Dose
• Start 300 mg 2–3 times/day and adjust dosage upward as indicated by plasma lithium levels

 Dosing Tips

✳ Sustained release formulation may reduce gastric irritation, lower peak lithium plasma levels, and diminish peak dose side effects (i.e., side effects occurring 1–2 hours after each dose of standard lithium carbonate may be improved by sustained release formulation)
• Lithium sulfate and other dosage strengths for lithium are available in Europe
• Check therapeutic blood levels as "trough" levels about 12 hours after the last dose
• After stabilization, some patients may do best with a once daily dose at night
• Responses in acute mania may take 7–14 days even with adequate plasma lithium levels
✳ Some patients apparently respond to doses as low as 300 mg twice a day, even with plasma lithium levels below 0.5 mEq/L
• Use the lowest dose of lithium associated with adequate therapeutic response
• Lower doses and lower plasma lithium levels (<0.6 mEq/L) are often adequate and advisable in the elderly
✳ Rapid discontinuation increases the risk of relapse and possibly suicide, so lithium

may need to be tapered slowly over 3 months if it is to be discontinued after long-term maintenance

Overdose
• Fatalities have occurred; tremor, dysarthria, delirium, coma, seizures, autonomic instability

Long-Term Use
• Indicated for long-term prevention of relapse
• May cause reduced kidney function
• Requires regular therapeutic monitoring of lithium levels as well as of kidney function and thyroid function

Habit Forming
• No

How to Stop
• Taper gradually over 3 months to avoid relapse
• Rapid discontinuation increases the risk of relapse, and possibly suicide
• Discontinuation symptoms uncommon

Pharmacokinetics
• Half life 18–30 hours

 Drug Interactions

✳ Non-steroidal anti-inflammatory agents, including ibuprofen and selective COX-2 inhibitors (cyclo-oxygenase 2), can increase plasma lithium concentrations; add with caution to patients stabilized on lithium
✳ Diuretics, especially thiazides, can increase plasma lithium concentrations; add with caution to patients stabilized on lithium
• Angiotensin-converting enzyme inhibitors can increase plasma lithium concentrations; add with caution to patients stabilized on lithium
• Metronidazole can lead to lithium toxicity through decreased renal clearance
• Acetazolamide, alkalizing agents, xanthine preparations, and urea may lower lithium plasma concentrations
• Methyldopa, carbamazepine, and phenytoin may interact with lithium to increase its toxicity

- Use lithium cautiously with calcium channel blockers, which may also increase lithium toxicity
- Use of lithium with an SSRI may raise risk of dizziness, confusion, diarrhea, agitation, tremor
- Some patients taking haloperidol and lithium have developed an encephalopathic syndrome similar to neuroleptic malignant syndrome
- Lithium may prolong effects of neuromuscular blocking agents
- No likely pharmacokinetic interactions of lithium with mood stabilizing anticonvulsants or atypical antipsychotics

 Other Warnings/ Precautions

✳ Toxic levels are near therapeutic levels; signs of toxicity include tremor, ataxia, diarrhea, vomiting, sedation
- Monitor for dehydration; lower dose if patient exhibits signs of infection, excessive sweating, diarrhea
- Closely monitor patients with thyroid disorders

Do Not Use

- If patient has severe kidney disease
- If patient has severe cardiovascular disease
- If patient has severe dehydration
- If patient has sodium depletion
- If there is a proven allergy to lithium

SPECIAL POPULATIONS

Renal Impairment

- Not recommended for use in patients with severe impairment

Hepatic Impairment

- No special indications

Cardiac Impairment

- Not recommended for use in patients with severe impairment

Elderly

- Likely that elderly patients will require lower doses to achieve therapeutic serum levels
- Elderly patients may be more sensitive to adverse effects

✳ Neurotoxicity, including delirium and other mental status changes, may occur even at therapeutic doses in elderly and organically compromised patients
- Lower doses and lower plasma lithium levels (<0.6 mEg/L) are often adequate and advisable in the elderly

 Children and Adolescents

- Safety and efficacy not established under age 12
- Use only with caution
- Younger children tend to have more frequent and severe side effects
- Children should be monitored more frequently

 Pregnancy

- Risk category D [positive evidence of risk to human fetus; potential benefits may still justify its use during pregnancy]
✳ Evidence of increased risk of major birth defects (perhaps 2–3 times the general population), but probably lower than with some other mood stabilizers (e.g., valproate)
- Evidence of increase in cardiac anomalies (especially Ebstein's anomaly) in infants whose mothers took lithium during pregnancy
- Lithium administration during delivery may be associated with hypotonia in the infant
- Use in women of childbearing potential requires weighing potential benefits to the mother against the risks to the fetus
- Taper drug if discontinuing
✳ For bipolar patients, lithium should generally be discontinued before anticipated pregnancies
- Recurrent bipolar illness during pregnancy can be quite disruptive
✳ For bipolar patients, given the risk of relapse in the postpartum period, lithium should generally be restarted immediately after delivery, but this generally means no breast feeding
✳ Atypical antipsychotics may be preferable to lithium or anticonvulsants if treatment of bipolar disorder is required during pregnancy

- Bipolar symptoms may recur or worsen during pregnancy and some form of treatment may be necessary

Breast Feeding

- Some drug is found in mother's breast milk, possibly at full therapeutic levels since lithium is soluble in breast milk
- ✳ Recommended either to discontinue drug or bottle feed
- ✳ Bipolar disorder may recur during the postpartum period, particularly if there is a history of prior postpartum episodes of either depression or psychosis
- ✳ Relapse rates may be lower in women who receive prophylactic treatment for postpartum episodes of bipolar disorder
- Atypical antipsychotics and anticonvulsants such as valproate may be safer than lithium during the postpartum period when breast feeding

THE ART OF PSYCHOPHARMACOLOGY

Potential Advantages

- Euphoric mania
- Treatment-resistant depression
- Reduces suicide risk
- Works well in combination with atypical antipsychotics and/or mood stabilizing anticonvulsants such as valproate

Potential Disadvantages

- Dysphoric mania
- Mixed mania, rapid-cycling mania
- Depressed phase of bipolar disorder
- Patients unable to tolerate weight gain, sedation, gastrointestinal effects, renal effects, and other side effects
- Requires blood monitoring

Primary Target Symptoms

- Unstable mood
- Mania

 Pearls

- ✳ Lithium was the original mood stabilizer and is still a first-line treatment option but may be underutilized since it is an older agent and is less promoted for use in bipolar disorder than newer agents

- ✳ May be best for euphoric mania; patients with rapid-cycling and mixed state types of bipolar disorder generally do less well on lithium
- ✳ Seems to be more effective in treating manic episodes than depressive episodes in bipolar disorder (treats from above better than it treats from below)
- ✳ May also be more effective in preventing manic relapses than in preventing depressive episodes (stabilizes from above better than it stabilizes from below)
- ✳ May decrease suicide and suicide attempts not only in bipolar I disorder but also in bipolar II disorder and in unipolar depression
- ✳ Due to its narrow therapeutic index, lithium's toxic side effects occur at doses close to its therapeutic effects
- Close therapeutic monitoring of plasma drug levels is required during lithium treatment; lithium is the first psychiatric drug that required blood level monitoring
- Probably less effective than atypical antipsychotics for severe, excited, disturbed, hyperactive, or psychotic patients with mania
- Due to delayed onset of action, lithium monotherapy may not be the first choice in acute mania, but rather may be used as an adjunct to atypical antipsychotics, benzodiazepines, and/or valproate loading
- After acute symptoms of mania are controlled, some patients can be maintained on lithium monotherapy
- However, only a third of bipolar patients experience adequate relief with a monotherapy, so most patients need multiple medications for best control
- Lithium is not a convincing augmentation agent to atypical antipsychotics for the treatment of schizophrenia
- Lithium is one of the most useful adjunctive agents to augment antidepressants for treatment-resistant unipolar depression
- Lithium may be useful for a number of patients with episodic, recurrent symptoms with or without affective illness, including episodic rage, anger or violence, and self-destructive behavior; such symptoms may be associated with psychotic or nonpsychotic illnesses, personality disorders, organic disorders, or mental retardation

- Lithium is better tolerated during acute manic phases than when manic symptoms have abated
- Adverse effects generally increase in incidence and severity as lithium serum levels increase
- Although not recommended for use in patients with severe renal or cardiovascular disease, dehydration, or sodium depletion, lithium can be administered cautiously in a hospital setting to such patients, with lithium serum levels determined daily
- Lithium-induced weight gain may be more common in women than in men

Suggested Reading

Delva NJ, Hawken ER. Preventing lithium intoxication. Guide for physicians. Can Fam Physician. 2001;47:1595–600.

Goodwin FK. Rationale for using lithium in combination with other mood stabilizers in the management of bipolar disorder. J Clin Psychiatry. 2003;64(Suppl 5):18–24.

Goodwin GM, Bowden CL, Calabrese JR et al. A pooled analysis of 2 placebo-controlled 18-month trials of lamotrigine and lithium maintenance treatment in bipolar I disorder. J Clin Psychiatry 2004;65:432–41.

Maj M. The effect of lithium in bipolar disorder: a review of recent research evidence. Bipolar Disord. 2003;5:180–8.

Tueth MJ, Murphy TK, Evans DL. Special considerations: use of lithium in children, adolescents, and elderly populations. J Clin Psychiatry. 1998;59 (Suppl 6):66–73.

OLANZAPINE

THERAPEUTICS

Brands
- Zyprexa
- Olasek
- Ziprexa
- Symbyax (olanzapine-fluoxetine combination)

see index for additional brand names

Generic? Not in U.S., Europe, or Japan

Class

- Atypical antipsychotic (serotonin-dopamine antagonist; second generation antipsychotic; also a mood stabilizer)

Commonly Prescribed For

(bold for FDA approved)
- **Schizophrenia**
- **Maintaining response in schizophrenia**
- **Acute agitation associated with schizophrenia (intramuscular)**
- **Acute mania/mixed mania (monotherapy and adjunct to lithium or valproate)**
- **Bipolar maintenance**
- **Acute agitation associated with bipolar I mania (intramuscular)**
- **Bipolar depression [in combination with fluoxetine (Symbyax)]**
- Other psychotic disorders
- Unipolar depression unresponsive to antidepressants
- Behavioral disturbances in dementias
- Behavioral disturbances in children and adolescents
- Disorders associated with problems with impulse control
- Borderline personality disorder

How The Drug Works

- Blocks dopamine 2 receptors, reducing positive symptoms of psychosis and stabilizing affective symptoms
- Blocks serotonin 2A receptors, causing enhancement of dopamine release in certain brain regions and thus reducing motor side effects and possibly improving cognitive and affective symptoms
- Interactions at a myriad of other neurotransmitter receptors may contribute to olanzapine's efficacy
- ✳ Specifically, antagonist actions at 5HT2C receptors may contribute to efficacy for cognitive and affective symptoms in some patients
- ✳ 5HT2C antagonist actions plus serotonin reuptake blockade of fluoxetine add to the actions of olanzapine when given as Symbyax (olanzapine-fluoxetine combination)

How Long Until It Works

- Psychotic and manic symptoms can improve within 1 week, but it may take several weeks for full effect on behavior as well as on cognition and affective stabilization
- Classically recommended to wait at least 4–6 weeks to determine efficacy of drug, but in practice some patients require up to 16–20 weeks to show a good response, especially on cognitive symptoms
- IM formulation can reduce agitation in 15–30 minutes

If It Works

- Most often reduces positive symptoms in schizophrenia but does not eliminate them
- Can improve negative symptoms, as well as aggressive, cognitive, and affective symptoms in schizophrenia
- Most schizophrenic patients do not have a total remission of symptoms but rather a reduction of symptoms by about a third
- Perhaps 5–15% of schizophrenic patients can experience an overall improvement of greater than 50–60%, especially when receiving stable treatment for more than a year
- Such patients are considered super-responders or "awakeners" since they may be well enough to be employed, live independently, and sustain long-term relationships
- Many bipolar patients may experience a reduction of symptoms by half or more
- Continue treatment until reaching a plateau of improvement
- After reaching a satisfactory plateau, continue treatment for at least a year after first episode of psychosis
- For second and subsequent episodes of psychosis, treatment may need to be indefinite
- Even for first episodes of psychosis, it may be preferable to continue treatment indefinitely to avoid subsequent episodes

- Treatment may not only reduce mania but also prevent recurrences of mania in bipolar disorder

If It Doesn't Work

- Try one of the other atypical antipsychotics (risperidone, quetiapine, ziprasidone, aripiprazole, amisulpride)
- If 2 or more antipsychotic monotherapies do not work, consider clozapine
- If no first-line atypical antipsychotic is effective, consider higher doses or augmentation with valproate or lamotrigine
- Some patients may require treatment with a conventional antipsychotic
- Consider noncompliance and switch to another antipsychotic with fewer side effects or to an antipsychotic that can be given by depot injection
- Consider initiating rehabilitation and psychotherapy
- Consider presence of concomitant drug abuse

Best Augmenting Combos for Partial Response or Treatment-Resistance

- Valproic acid (valproate, divalproex, divalproex ER)
- Other mood stabilizing anticonvulsants (carbamazepine, oxcarbazepine, lamotrigine)
- Lithium
- Benzodiazepines
- Fluoxetine and other antidepressants may be effective augmenting agents to olanzapine for bipolar depression, psychotic depression, and for unipolar depression not responsive to antidepressants alone (e.g., olanzapine-fluoxetine combination)

Tests

Before starting an atypical antipsychotic

✷ Weigh all patients and track BMI during treatment
- Get baseline personal and family history of diabetes, obesity, dyslipidemia, hypertension, and cardiovascular disease
✷ Get waist circumference (at umbilicus), blood pressure, fasting plasma glucose, and fasting lipid profile
- Determine if the patient is
  - overweight (BMI 25.0–29.9)

  - obese (BMI ≥30)
  - has pre-diabetes (fasting plasma glucose 100–125 mg/dl)
  - has diabetes (fasting plasma glucose >126 mg/dl)
  - has hypertension (BP >140/90 mm Hg)
  - has dyslipidemia (increased total cholesterol, LDL cholesterol, and triglycerides; decreased HDL cholesterol)
- Treat or refer such patients for treatment, including nutrition and weight management, physical activity counseling, smoking cessation, and medical management

Monitoring after starting an atypical antipsychotic

✷ BMI monthly for 3 months, then quarterly
✷ Blood pressure, fasting plasma glucose, fasting lipids within 3 months and then annually, but earlier and more frequently for patients with diabetes or who have gained >5% of initial weight
- Treat or refer for treatment and consider switching to another atypical antipsychotic for patients who become overweight, obese, pre-diabetic, diabetic, hypertensive, or dyslipidemic while receiving an atypical antipsychotic
✷ Even in patients without known diabetes, be vigilant for the rare but life threatening onset of diabetic ketoacidosis, which always requires immediate treatment, by monitoring for the rapid onset of polyuria, polydipsia, weight loss, nausea, vomiting, dehydration, rapid respiration, weakness and clouding of sensorium, even coma
- Patients with liver disease should have blood tests a few times a year

SIDE EFFECTS

How Drug Causes Side Effects

- By blocking histamine 1 receptors in the brain, it can cause sedation and possibly weight gain
- By blocking alpha 1 adrenergic receptors, it can cause dizziness, sedation, and hypotension
- By blocking muscarinic 1 receptors, it can cause dry mouth, constipation, and sedation

- By blocking dopamine 2 receptors in the striatum, it can cause motor side effects (unusual)
- Mechanism of weight gain and increased incidence of diabetes and dyslipidemia with atypical antipsychotics is unknown but insulin regulation may be impaired by blocking pancreatic M3 muscarinic receptors

Notable Side Effects

✳ Probably increases risk for diabetes mellitus and dyslipidemia
- Dizziness, sedation
- Dry mouth, constipation, dyspepsia, weight gain
- Peripheral edema
- Joint pain, back pain, chest pain, extremity pain, abnormal gait, ecchymosis
- Tachycardia
- Orthostatic hypotension, usually during initial dose titration
- Rare tardive dyskinesia (much reduced risk compared to conventional antipsychotics)
- Rare rash on exposure to sunlight

 ## Life Threatening or Dangerous Side Effects

- Hyperglycemia, in some cases extreme and associated with ketoacidosis or hyperosmolar coma or death, has been reported in patients taking atypical antipsychotics
- Rare neuroleptic malignant syndrome (much reduced risk compared to conventional antipsychotics)
- Rare seizures
- Increased risk of death and cerebrovascular events in elderly patients with dementia-related psychosis

Weight Gain

- Frequent and can be significant in amount
- Can become a health problem in some
- More than for some other antipsychotics, but never say always as not a problem in everyone

Sedation

- Many patients experience and/or can be significant in amount
- Usually transient
- May be less than for some antipsychotics, more than for others

What To Do About Side Effects

- Wait
- Wait
- Wait
- Take at bedtime to help reduce daytime sedation
- Anticholinergics may reduce motor side effects such as akathisia when present, but rarely necessary
- Weight loss, exercise programs, and medical management for high BMIs, diabetes, dyslipidemia
- Switch to another atypical antipsychotic

Best Augmenting Agents for Side Effects

- Benztropine or trihexyphenidyl for motor side effects
- Many side effects cannot be improved with an augmenting agent

DOSING AND USE

Usual Dosage Range

- 10–20 mg/day (oral or intramuscular)
- 6–12 mg olanzapine / 25–50 mg fluoxetine (olanzapine-fluoxetine combination)

Dosage Forms

- Tablets 2.5 mg, 5 mg, 7.5 mg, 10 mg, 15 mg, 20 mg
- Orally disintegrating tablets 5 mg, 10 mg, 15 mg, 20 mg
- Intramuscular formulation 5 mg/mL, each vial contains 10 mg (available in some countries)
- Olanzapine-fluoxetine combination capsule (mg equivalent olanzapine/mg equivalent fluoxetine) 6 mg/25 mg, 6 mg/50 mg, 12 mg/25 mg, 12 mg/50 mg

How to Dose

- Initial 5–10 mg once daily orally; increase by 5 mg/day once a week until desired efficacy is reached; maximum approved dose is 20 mg/day
- For intramuscular formulation, recommended initial dose 10 mg; second

injection of 5–10 mg may be administered 2 hours after first injection; maximum daily dose of olanzapine is 20 mg, with no more than 3 injections per 24 hours

- For olanzapine-fluoxetine combination, recommended initial dose 6 mg/25 mg once daily in evening; increase dose based on efficacy and tolerability; maximum generally 18 mg/75 mg

 Dosing Tips

✻ **More may be more:** raising usual dose above 15 mg/day can be useful for acutely ill and agitated patients and some treatment-resistant patients, gaining efficacy without many more side effects

✻ Some heroic uses for patients who do not respond to other antipsychotics can occasionally justify dosing over 30 mg/day

- Usual doses (>15 mg/day range) can be among the most costly among atypical antipsychotics, and dosing >30 mg/day can be very expensive
- Rather than raise the dose above these levels in acutely agitated patients requiring acute antipsychotic actions, consider augmentation with a benzodiazepine or conventional antipsychotic, either orally or intramuscularly
- Rather than raise the dose above these levels in partial responders, consider augmentation with a mood stabilizing anticonvulsant, such as valproate or lamotrigine
- Clearance of olanzapine is slightly reduced in women compared to men, so women may need lower doses than men
- Children and elderly should generally be dosed at the lower end of the dosage spectrum

✻ Olanzapine intramuscularly can be given short-term, both to initiate dosing with oral olanzapine or another oral antipsychotic and to treat breakthrough agitation in patients maintained on oral antipsychotics

Overdose

- Rarely lethal in monotherapy overdose; sedation, slurred speech

Long-Term Use

- Approved to maintain response in long-term treatment of schizophrenia

- Approved for long-term maintenance in bipolar disorder
- Often used for long-term maintenance in various behavioral disorders

Habit Forming

- No

How to Stop

- Slow down-titration of oral formulation (over 6 to 8 weeks), especially when simultaneously beginning a new antipsychotic while switching (i.e., cross-titration)
- Rapid oral discontinuation may lead to rebound psychosis and worsening of symptoms

Pharmacokinetics

- Metabolites are inactive
- Parent drug has 21–54 hour half-life

 Drug Interactions

- May increase effect of anti-hypertensive agents
- May antagonize levodopa, dopamine agonists
- Dose may need to be lowered if given with CYP450 1A2 inhibitors (e.g., fluvoxamine); raised if given in conjunction with CYP450 1A2 inducers (e.g., cigarette smoke, carbamazepine)

 Other Warnings/ Precautions

- Use with caution in patients with conditions that predispose to hypotension (dehydration, overheating)
- Use with caution in patients with prostatic hypertrophy, narrow angle-closure glaucoma, paralytic ileus
- Patients receiving the intramuscular formulation of olanzapine should be observed closely for hypotension
- Intramuscular formulation is not generally recommended to be administered with parenteral benzodiazepines; if patient requires a parenteral benzodiazepine it should be given at least 1 hour after intramuscular olanzapine
- Olanzapine should be used cautiously in patients at risk for aspiration pneumonia, as dysphagia has been reported

Do Not Use
- If there is a known risk of narrow angle-closure glaucoma (intramuscular formulation)
- If patient has unstable medical condition (e.g., acute myocardial infarction, unstable angina pectoris, severe hypotension and/or bradycardia, sick sinus syndrome, recent heart surgery) (intramuscular formulation)
- If there is a proven allergy to olanzapine

SPECIAL POPULATIONS

Renal Impairment
- No dose adjustment required for oral formulation
- Not removed by hemodialysis
- For intramuscular formulation, consider lower starting dose (5 mg)

Hepatic Impairment
- May need to lower dose
- Patients with liver disease should have liver function tests a few times a year
- For moderate to severe hepatic impairment, starting oral dose 5 mg; increase with caution
- For intramuscuar formulation, consider lower starting dose (5 mg)

Cardiac Impairment
- Drug should be used with caution because of risk of orthostatic hypotension

Elderly
- Some patients may tolerate lower doses better
- Increased incidence of stroke
- For intramuscular formulation, recommended starting dose is 2.5–5 mg; a second injection of 2.5–5 mg may be administered 2 hours after first injection; no more than 3 injections should be administered within 24 hours
- Although atypical antipsychotics are commonly used for behavioral disturbances in dementia, no agent has been approved for treatment of elderly patients with dementia-related psychosis
- Elderly patients with dementia-related psychosis treated with atypical antipsychotics are at an increased risk of death compared to placebo, and also have an increased risk of cerebrovascular events

Children and Adolescents
- Not officially recommended under age 18; however, olanzapine is often used for patients under 18
- Clinical experience and early data suggest olanzapine is probably safe and effective for behavioral disturbances in children and adolescents
- Children and adolescents using olanzapine may need to be monitored more often than adults
- Intramuscular formulation has not been studied in patients under 18 and is not recommended for use in this population

Pregnancy
- Risk Category C [some animal studies show adverse effects, no controlled studies in humans]
- Psychotic symptoms may worsen during pregnancy, and some form of treatment may be necessary
- Early findings of infants exposed to olanzapine in utero currently do not show adverse consequences
- Olanzapine may be preferable to anticonvulsant mood stabilizers if treatment is required during pregnancy

Breast Feeding
- Unknown if olanzapine is secreted in human breast milk, but all psychotropics assumed to be secreted in breast milk
- ✳ Recommended either to discontinue drug or bottle feed
- Infants of women who choose to breast feed while on olanzapine should be monitored for possible adverse effects

THE ART OF PSYCHOPHARMACOLOGY

Potential Advantages
- ✳ Some cases of psychosis and bipolar disorder refractory to treatment with other antipsychotics
- ✳ Often a preferred augmenting agent in bipolar depression or treatment-resistant unipolar depression
- ✳ Patients needing rapid onset of antipsychotic action without drug titration

- Patients switching from intramuscular olanzapine to an oral preparation

Potential Disadvantages

- Patients concerned about gaining weight
- ✻ Patients with diabetes mellitus, obesity, and/or dyslipidemia

Primary Target Symptoms

- Positive symptoms of psychosis
- Negative symptoms of psychosis
- Cognitive symptoms
- Unstable mood (both depressed mood and mania)
- Aggressive symptoms

Pearls

- Recent landmark head to head study in schizophrenia suggests greater effectiveness (i.e., lower dropouts of all causes) at moderately high doses compared to some other atypical and conventional antipsychotics at moderate doses
- Same recent head to head study in schizophrenia suggests greater efficacy but greater metabolic side effects compared to some other atypical and conventional antipsychotics
- Well accepted for use in schizophrenia and bipolar disorder, including difficult cases
- ✻ Documented utility in treatment-refractory cases, especially at higher doses
- ✻ Documented efficacy as augmenting agent to SSRIs (fluoxetine) in nonpsychotic treatment-resistant major depressive disorder
- ✻ Documented efficacy in bipolar depression, especially in combination with fluoxetine
- More weight gain than many other antipsychotics —does not mean every patient gains weight
- Motor side effects unusual at low- to mid-doses
- Less sedation than for some other antipsychotics, more than for others
- ✻ Controversial as to whether olanzapine has more risk of diabetes and dyslipidemia than other antipsychotics
- One of the most expensive atypical antipsychotics within the usual therapeutic dosing range
- Cigarette smoke can decrease olanzapine levels and patients may require a dose increase if they begin or increase smoking
- ✻ One of only two atypical antipsychotics with a short-acting intramuscular dosage formulation

Suggested Reading

Duggan L, Fenton M, Dardennes RM, El-Dosoky A, Indran S. Olanzapine for schizophrenia. Cochrane Database Syst Rev 2003;(1):CD001359.

Kapur S, Remington G. Atypical antipsychotics: new directions and new challenges in the treatment of schizophrenia. Annu Rev Med 2001;52:503–17.

Lieberman JA, Stroup TS, McEvoy JP, Swartz MS, Rosenheck RA, Perkins DO et al. Effectiveness of antipsychotic drugs in patients with chronic schizophrenia. N Engl J Med 2005;353(12):1209–23.

Tandon R. Safety and tolerability: how do new generation "atypical" antipsychotics compare? Psychiatric Quarterly 2002;73:297–311.

Tandon R, Jibson MD. Efficacy of newer generation antipsychotics in the treatment of schizophrenia. Psychoneuroendocrinology 2003;28:9–26.

Yatham LN. Efficacy of atypical antipsychotics in mood disorders. J Clin Psychopharmacol 2003;23(3 Suppl 1):S9–14.

OXCARBAZEPINE

THERAPEUTICS

Brands • Trileptal
see index for additional brand names

Generic? No

Class
• Anticonvulsant, voltage-sensitive sodium channel antagonist

Commonly Prescribed For
(bold for FDA approved)
• **Partial seizures in adults with epilepsy (monotherapy or adjunctive)**
• **Partial seizures in children ages 4–16 with epilepsy (monotherapy or adjunctive)**
• Bipolar disorder

How The Drug Works
✳ Acts as a use-dependent blocker of voltage-sensitive sodium channels
✳ Interacts with the open channel conformation of voltage-sensitive sodium channels
✳ Interacts at a specific site of the alpha pore-forming subunit of voltage-sensitive sodium channels
• Inhibits release of glutamate

How Long Until It Works
• For acute mania, effects should occur within a few weeks
• May take several weeks to months to optimize an effect on mood stabilization
• Should reduce seizures by 2 weeks

If It Works
• The goal of treatment is complete remission of symptoms (e.g., seizures, mania)
• Continue treatment until all symptoms are gone or until improvement is stable and then continue treating indefinitely as long as improvement persists
• Continue treatment indefinitely to avoid recurrence of mania and seizures

If It Doesn't Work (for bipolar disorder)
✳ Many patients only have a partial response where some symptoms are improved but others persist or continue to wax and wane without stabilization of mood
• Other patients may be nonresponders, sometimes called treatment-resistant or treatment-refractory
• Consider increasing dose, switching to another agent or adding an appropriate augmenting agent
• Consider adding psychotherapy
• For bipolar disorder, consider the presence of noncompliance and counsel patient
• Switch to another mood stabilizer with fewer side effects
• Consider evaluation for another diagnosis or for a comorbid condition (e.g., medical illness, substance abuse, etc.)

Best Augmenting Combos for Partial Response or Treatment-Resistance
• Oxcarbazepine is itself a second-line augmenting agent for numerous other anticonvulsants, lithium, and atypical antipsychotics in treating bipolar disorder, although its use in bipolar disorder is not yet well-studied
• Oxcarbazepine may be a second or third-line augmenting agent for antipsychotics in treating schizophrenia, although its use in schizophrenia is also not yet well-studied

Tests
• Consider monitoring sodium levels because of possibility of hyponatremia, especially during the first 3 months

SIDE EFFECTS

How Drug Causes Side Effects
• CNS side effects theoretically due to excessive actions at voltage-sensitive sodium channels

Notable Side Effects
✳ Sedation, dizziness, headache, ataxia, nystagmus, abnormal gait, confusion, nervousness, fatigue
✳ Nausea, vomiting, abdominal pain, dyspepsia
• Diplopia, vertigo, abnormal vision
✳ Rash

Life Threatening or Dangerous Side Effects
- Hyponatremia

Weight Gain

unusual | not unusual | common | problematic

- Occurs in significant minority
- Some patients experience increased appetite

Sedation

unusual | not unusual | common | problematic

- Occurs in significant minority
- Dose-related
- Less than carbamazepine
- More when combined with other anticonvulsants
- Can wear off with time, but may not wear off at high doses

What To Do About Side Effects
- Wait
- Wait
- Wait
- Switch to another agent

Best Augmenting Agents for Side Effects
- Many side effects cannot be improved with an augmenting agent

DOSING AND USE

Usual Dosage Range
- 1200–2400 mg/day

Dosage Forms
- Tablet 150 mg, 300 mg, 600 mg
- Liquid 300 mg/5 mL

How to Dose
- Monotherapy for seizures or bipolar disorder: initial 600 mg/day in 2 doses; increase every 3 days by 300 mg/day; maximum dose generally 2400 mg/day
- Adjunctive: initial 600 mg/day in 2 doses; each week can increase by 600 mg/day; recommended dose 1200 mg/day; maximum dose generally 2400 mg/day

- When converting from adjunctive to monotherapy in the treatment of epilepsy, titrate concomitant drug down over 3–6 weeks while titrating oxcarbazepine up over 2–4 weeks, with an initial daily oxcarbazepine dose of 600 mg divided in 2 doses

 Dosing Tips
- ✱ Doses of oxcarbazepine need to be about one-third higher than those of carbamazepine for similar results
- Usually administered as adjunctive medication to other anticonvulsants, lithium, or atypical antipsychotics for bipolar disorder
- Side effects may increase with dose
- Although increased efficacy for seizures is seen at 2400 mg/day compared to 1200 mg/day, CNS side effects may be intolerable at the higher dose
- Liquid formulation can be administered mixed in a glass of water or directly from the oral dosing syringe supplied
- Slow dose titration may delay onset of therapeutic action but enhance tolerability to sedating side effects
- Should titrate slowly in the presence of other sedating agents, such as other anticonvulsants, in order to best tolerate additive sedative side effects

Overdose
- No fatalities reported

Long-Term Use
- Safe
- Monitoring of sodium may be required, especially during the first 3 months

Habit Forming
- No

How to Stop
- Taper
- Epilepsy patients may seize upon withdrawal, especially if withdrawal is abrupt
- ✱ Rapid discontinuation may increase the risk of relapse in bipolar disorder
- Discontinuation symptoms uncommon

Pharmacokinetics
- Metabolized in the liver

- Renally excreted
- Inhibits CYP450 2C19
* Oxcarbazepine is a prodrug for 10-hydroxy carbazepine
* This main active metabolite is sometimes called the monohydroxy derivative or MHD, and is also known as licarbazepine
* Half-life of parent drug is approximately 2 hours; half-life of MHD is approximately 9 hours; thus oxcarbazepine is essentially a prodrug rapidly converted to its MHD, licarbazepine
- A mild inducer of CYP450 3A4

Drug Interactions

- Depressive effects may be increased by other CNS depressants (alcohol, MAOIs, other anticonvulsants, etc.)
- Strong inducers of CYP450 cytochromes (e.g., carbamazepine, phenobarbital, phenytoin, and primidone) can decrease plasma levels of the active metabolite MHD
- Verapamil may decrease plasma levels of the active metabolite MHD
- Oxcarbazepine can decrease plasma levels of hormonal contraceptives and dihydropyridine calcium antagonists
- Oxcarbazepine at doses greater than 1200 mg/day may increase plasma levels of phenytoin, possibly requiring dose reduction of phenytoin

Other Warnings/ Precautions

- Because oxcarbazepine has a tricyclic chemical structure, it is not recommended to be taken with MAOIs, including 14 days after MAOIs are stopped; do not start an MAOI until 2 weeks after discontinuing oxcarbazepine
- Because oxcarbazepine can lower plasma levels of hormonal contraceptives, it may also reduce their effectiveness
- May exacerbate narrow angle-closure glaucoma
- May need to restrict fluids and/or monitor sodium because of risk of hyponatremia
- Use cautiously in patients who have demonstrated hypersensitivity to carbamazepine

Do Not Use

- If patient is taking an MAOI

- If there is a proven allergy to any tricyclic compound
- If there is a proven allergy to oxcarbazepine

SPECIAL POPULATIONS

Renal Impairment

- Oxcarbazepine is renally excreted
- Elimination half-life of active metabolite MHD is increased
- Reduce initial dose by half; may need to use slower titration

Hepatic Impairment

- No dose adjustment recommended for mild to moderate hepatic impairment

Cardiac Impairment

- No dose adjustment recommended

Elderly

- Older patients may have reduced creatinine clearance and require reduced dosing
- Elderly patients may be more susceptible to adverse effects
- Some patients may tolerate lower doses better

Children and Adolescents

- Approved as adjunctive therapy or monotherapy for partial seizures in children 4 and older
- Ages 4–16 (adjunctive): initial 8–10 mg/kg/day or less than 600 mg/day in 2 doses; increase over 2 weeks to 900 mg/day (20–29 kg), 1200 mg/day (29.1–39 kg), or 1800 mg/day (>39 kg)
- When converting from adjunctive to monotherapy, titrate concomitant drug down over 3–6 weeks while titrating oxcarbazepine up by no more than 10 mg/kg/day each week, with an initial daily oxcarbazepine dose of 8–10 mg/kg/day divided in 2 doses
- Monotherapy: Initial 8–10 mg/kg/day in 2 doses; increase every 3 days by 5 mg/kg/day; recommended maintenance dose dependent on weight
- 0–20 kg (600–900 mg/day); 21–30 kg (900–1200 mg/day); 31–40 kg (900–1500 mg/day);

41–45 kg (1200–1500 mg/day);
46–55 kg (1200–1800 mg/day);
56–65 kg (1200–2100 mg/day);
over 65 kg (1500–2100 mg)

• Children below age 8 may have increased clearance compared to adults

Pregnancy

• Risk category C [some animal studies show adverse effects, no controlled studies in humans]
✳ Oxcarbazepine is structurally similar to carbamazepine, which is thought to be teratogenic in humans
✳ Use during first trimester may raise risk of neural tube defects (e.g., spina bifida) or other congenital anomalies
• Use in women of childbearing potential requires weighing potential benefits to the mother against the risks to the fetus
✳ If drug is continued, perform tests to detect birth defects
✳ If drug is continued, start on folate 1 mg/day to reduce risk of neural tube defects
• Antiepileptic Drug Pregnancy Registry: (888) 233-2334
• Taper drug if discontinuing
✳ For bipolar patients, oxcarbazepine should generally be discontinued before anticipated pregnancies
• Seizures, even mild seizures, may cause harm to the embryo/fetus
• Recurrent bipolar illness during pregnancy can be quite disruptive
✳ For bipolar patients, given the risk of relapse in the postpartum period, some form of mood stabilizer treatment may need to be restarted immediately after delivery if patient is unmedicated during pregnancy
✳ Atypical antipsychotics may be preferable to lithium or anticonvulsants such as oxcarbazepine if treatment of bipolar disorder is required during pregnancy
• Bipolar symptoms may recur or worsen during pregnancy and some form of treatment may be necessary

Breast Feeding

• Some drug is found in mother's breast milk
✳ Recommended either to discontinue drug or bottle feed

• If drug is continued while breast feeding, infant should be monitored for possible adverse effects
• If infant shows signs of irritability or sedation, drug may need to be discontinued
• Bipolar disorder may recur during the postpartum period, particularly if there is a history of prior postpartum episodes of either depression or psychosis
✳ Relapse rates may be lower in women who receive prophylactic treatment for postpartum episodes of bipolar disorder
• Atypical antipsychotics and anticonvulsants such as valproate may be safer than oxcarbazepine during the postpartum period when breast feeding

THE ART OF PSYCHOPHARMACOLOGY

Potential Advantages
• Treatment-resistant bipolar and psychotic disorders
• Those unable to tolerate carbamazepine but who respond to carbamazepine

Potential Disadvantages
• Patients at risk for hyponatremia

Primary Target Symptoms
• Incidence of seizures
• Severity of seizures
• Unstable mood, especially mania

Pearls
✳ Some evidence of effectiveness in treating acute mania; included in American Psychiatric Association's bipolar treatment guidelines as an option for acute treatment and maintenance treatment of bipolar disorder
• Some evidence of effectiveness as adjunctive treatment in schizophrenia and schizoaffective disorders
• Oxcarbazepine is the 10-keto analog of carbamazepine, but not a metabolite of carbamazepine
• Less well investigated in bipolar disorder than carbamazepine
✳ Oxcarbazepine seems to have the same mechanism of therapeutic action as carbamazepine but with fewer side effects

✹ Specifically, risk of leukopenia, aplastic anemia, agranulocytosis, elevated liver enzymes, or Stevens Johnson syndrome and serious rash associated with carbamazepine does <u>not</u> seem to be associated with oxcarbazepine

• Skin rash reactions to carbamazepine may resolve in 75% of patients with epilepsy when switched to oxcarbazepine; thus, 25% of patients who experience rash with carbamazepine may also experience it with oxcarbazepine

• Oxcarbazepine has much less prominent actions on CYP 450 enzyme systems than carbamazepine, and thus fewer drug-drug interactions

• Specifically, oxcarbazepine and its active metabolite, the monohydroxy derivative (MHD), cause less enzyme induction of CYP450 3A4 than the structurally-related carbamazepine

• The active metabolite MHD, also called licarbazepine, is a racemic mixture of 80% S-MHD (active) and 20% R-MHD (inactive)

• R, S-licarbazepine is also in clinical development as a novel mood stabilizer

• The active S enantiomer of licarbazepine is another related compound in development as yet another novel mood stabilizer

✹ Most significant risk of oxcarbazepine may be clinically significant hyponatremia (sodium level <125 m mol/L), most likely occurring within the first 3 months of treatment, and occurring in 2–3% of patients

• Unknown if this risk is higher than for carbamazepine

✹ Since SSRIs can sometimes also reduce sodium due to SIADH (syndrome of inappropriate antidiuretic hormone production), patients treated with combinations of oxcarbazepine and SSRIs should be carefully monitored, especially in the early stages of treatment

• By analogy with carbamazepine, could theoretically be useful in chronic neuropathic pain

Suggested Reading

Beydoun A. Safety and efficacy of oxcarbazepine: results of randomized, double-blind trials. Pharmacotherapy. 2000; 20(8 Pt 2):152S–158S.

Centorrino F, Albert MJ, Berry JM, Kelleher JP, Fellman V, Line G, Koukopoulos AE, Kidwell JE, Fogarty KV, Baldessarini RJ. Oxcarbazepine: clinical experience with hospitalized psychiatric patients. Bipolar Disord. 2003;5:370–4.

Dietrich DE, Kropp S, Emrich HM. Oxcarbazepine in affective and schizoaffective disorders. Pharmacopsychiatry. 2001;34:242–50.

Glauser TA. Oxcarbazepine in the treatment of epilepsy. Pharmacotherapy. 2001;21:904–19.

Hellewell JS. Oxcarbazepine (Trileptal) in the treatment of bipolar disorders: a review of efficacy and tolerability. J Affect Disord. 2002;72(Suppl 1):S23–34.

PEROSPIRONE

THERAPEUTICS

Brands • Lullan
see index for additional brand names

Generic? No

Class

• Atypical antipsychotic (serotonin-dopamine antagonist, second generation antipsychotic)

Commonly Prescribed For
(bold for FDA approved)
• Schizophrenia (Japan)

How The Drug Works

• Blocks dopamine 2 receptors, reducing positive symptoms of psychosis
• Blocks serotonin 2A receptors, causing enhancement of dopamine release in certain brain regions and thus reducing motor side effects and possibly improving cognitive and affective symptoms
✷ Interactions at 5HT1A receptors may contribute to efficacy for cognitive and affective symptoms in some patients

How Long Until It Works

• Psychotic symptoms can improve within 1 week, but it may take several weeks for full effect on behavior as well as on cognition and affective stabilization
• Classically recommended to wait at least 4–6 weeks to determine efficacy of drug, but in practice some patients require up to 16–20 weeks to show a good response, especially on cognitive symptoms

If It Works

• Most often reduces positive symptoms in schizophrenia but does not eliminate them
• Can improve negative symptoms, as well as aggressive, cognitive, and affective symptoms in schizophrenia
• Most schizophrenic patients do not have a total remission of symptoms but rather a reduction of symptoms by about a third
• Perhaps 5–15% of schizophrenic patients can experience an overall improvement of greater than 50–60%, especially when receiving stable treatment for more than a year

• Such patients are considered super-responders or "awakeners" since they may be well enough to be employed, live independently, and sustain long-term relationships
• Continue treatment until reaching a plateau of improvement
• After reaching a satisfactory plateau, continue treatment for at least a year after first episode of psychosis
• For second and subsequent episodes of psychosis, treatment may need to be indefinite
• Even for first episodes of psychosis, it may be preferable to continue treatment

If It Doesn't Work

• Consider trying one of the first-line atypical antipsychotics (e.g. risperidone, olanzapine, quetiapine, aripiprazole)
• If 2 or more antipsychotic monotherapies do not work, consider clozapine
• If no first-line atypical antipsychotic is effective, consider higher doses or augmentation with valproate or lamotrigine
• Some patients may require treatment with a conventional antipsychotic
• Consider noncompliance and switch to another antipsychotic with fewer side effects or to an antipsychotic that can be given by depot injection
• Consider initiating rehabilitation and psychotherapy
• Consider presence of concomitant drug abuse

Best Augmenting Combos for Partial Response or Treatment-Resistance

• Augmentation of perospirone has not been systematically studied
• Addition of a benzodiazepine, especially short-term for agitation
• Addition of a mood stabilizing anticonvulsant such as valproate, carbamazepine, or lamotrigine may theoretically be helpful in both schizophrenia and bipolar mania
• Augmentation with lithium in bipolar mania may be helpful

Tests

✷ Potential of weight gain, diabetes, and dyslipidemia associated with perospirone has not been systematically studied, but patients should be monitored the same as for other atypical antipsychotics

Before starting an atypical antipsychotic

✳ Weigh all patients and track BMI during treatment
• Get baseline personal and family history of diabetes, obesity, dyslipidemia, hypertension, and cardiovascular disease
✳ Get waist circumference (at umbilicus), blood pressure, fasting plasma glucose, and fasting lipid profile
• Determine if patient is
  • overweight (BMI 25.0–29.9)
  • obese (BMI ≥30)
  • has pre-diabetes (fasting plasma glucose 100–125 mg/dl)
  • has diabetes (fasting plasma glucose >126 mg/dl)
  • has hypertension (BP >140/90 mm Hg)
  • has dyslipidemia (increased total cholesterol, LDL cholesterol, and triglycerides; decreased HDL cholesterol)
• Treat or refer such patients for treatment, including nutrition and weight management, physical activity counseling, smoking cessation, and medical management

Monitoring after starting an atypical antipsychotic

✳ BMI monthly for 3 months, then quarterly
✳ Blood pressure, fasting plasma glucose, fasting lipids within 3 months and then annually, but earlier and more frequently for patients with diabetes or who have gained >5% of initial weight
• Treat or refer for treatment and consider switching to another atypical antipsychotic for patients who become overweight, obese, pre-diabetic, diabetic, hypertensive, or dyslipidemic while receiving an atypical antipsychotic
✳ Even in patients without known diabetes, be vigilant for the rare but life threatening onset of diabetic ketoacidosis, which always requires immediate treatment, by monitoring for the rapid onset of polyuria, polydipsia, weight loss, nausea, vomiting, dehydration, rapid respiration, weakness and clouding of sensorium, even coma
• Should check blood pressure in the elderly before starting and for the first few weeks of treatment

SIDE EFFECTS

How Drug Causes Side Effects

• By blocking dopamine 2 receptors in the striatum, it can cause motor side effects
• By blocking dopamine 2 receptors in the pituitary, it can cause increased prolactin (unusual)
• Mechanism of weight gain and increased incidence of diabetes and dyslipidemia with some atypical antipsychotics is unknown
• Receptor binding portfolio of perospirone is not well-characterized

Notable Side Effects

✳ Extrapyramidal symptoms, akathisia
✳ Insomnia
• Sedation, anxiety, weakness, headache, anorexia, constipation
• Theoretically, tardive dyskinesia (should be reduced risk compared to conventional antipsychotics)
• Elevated creatine phosphokinase levels

 Life Threatening or Dangerous Side Effects

• Rare neuroleptic malignant syndrome
• Theoretically, seizures are rarely associated with atypical antipsychotics
• Increased risk of death and cerebrovascular events in elderly patients with dementia-related psychosis

Weight Gain

✳ Not well characterized

Sedation

unusual   not unusual   common   problematic

• Occurs in significant minority

What To Do About Side Effects

• Wait
• Wait
• Wait
• For motor symptoms, add an anticholinergic agent
• Reduce the dose
• Switch to another atypical antipsychotic

Best Augmenting Agents for Side Effects

• Benztropine or trihexyphenidyl for motor side effects

- Sometimes amantadine can be helpful for motor side effects
- Benzodiazepines may be helpful for akathisia
- Many side effects cannot be improved with an augmenting agent

DOSING AND USE

Usual Dosage Range
- 8–48 mg/day in 3 divided doses

Dosage Forms
- Tablet 4 mg, 8 mg

How to Dose
- Begin at 4 mg 3 times a day, increasing as tolerated up to 16 mg 3 times a day

 Dosing Tips
- Some patients have been treated with up to 96 mg/day in 3 divided doses
- Unknown whether dosing frequency can be reduced to once or twice daily, but by analogy with other agents in this class with half-lives shorter than 24 hours, this may be possible

Overdose
- Not reported

Long-Term Use
- Long-term studies not reported, but as for other atypical antipsychotics, long-term use for treatment of schizophrenia is common

Habit Forming
- No

How to Stop
- Slow down-titration (over 6 to 8 weeks), especially when simultaneously beginning a new antipsychotic while switching (i.e., cross-titration)
- Rapid discontinuation may lead to rebound psychosis and worsening of symptoms
- If antiparkinson agents are being used, they should be continued for a few weeks after perospirone is discontinued

Pharmacokinetics
- Metabolized primarily by CYP450 3A4

- No active metabolites

 Drug Interactions
- Ketoconazole and possibly other CYP450 3A4 inhibitors such as nefazodone, fluvoxamine, and fluoxetine may increase plasma levels of perospirone
- Carbamazepine and possibly other inducers of CYP450 3A4 may decrease plasma levels of perospirone

 Other Warnings/ Precautions
- Not reported

Do Not Use
- If there is a proven allergy to perospirone

SPECIAL POPULATIONS

Renal Impairment
- Use with caution

Hepatic Impairment
- Use with caution

Cardiac Impairment
- Use with caution

Elderly
- Some patients may tolerate lower doses better
- Although atypical antipsychotics are commonly used for behavioral disturbances in dementia, no agent has been approved for treatment of elderly patients with dementia-related psychosis
- Elderly patients with dementia-related psychosis treated with atypical antipsychotics are at an increased risk of death compared to placebo, and also have an increased risk of cerebrovascular events

 Children and Adolescents
- Use with caution

Pregnancy

- Psychotic symptoms may worsen during pregnancy and some form of treatment may be necessary

Breast Feeding

- Unknown if perospirone is secreted in human breast milk, but all psychotropics assumed to be secreted in breast milk
- ✳ Recommended either to discontinue drug or bottle feed
- Infants of women who choose to breast feed should be monitored for possible adverse effects

THE ART OF PSYCHOPHARMACOLOGY

Potential Advantages

- In Japan, studies suggest efficacy for negative symptoms of schizophrenia

Potential Disadvantages

- Patients who have difficulty complying with three times daily administration

Primary Target Symptoms

- Positive symptoms of psychosis
- Negative symptoms of psychosis
- Affective symptoms (depression, anxiety)
- Cognitive symptoms

 Pearls

- Extrapyramidal symptoms may be more frequent than with some other atypical antipsychotics
- Potent 5HT1A binding properties may be helpful for improving cognitive symptoms of schizophrenia in long-term treatment
- Theoretically, should be effective in acute bipolar mania

 Suggested Reading

Ohno Y. Pharmacological characteristics of perospirone hydrochloride, a novel antipsychotic agent. Nippon Yakurigaku Zasshi 2000; 116 (4): 225–31.

PREGABALIN

THERAPEUTICS

Brands • Lyrica
see index for additional brand names

Generic? No

 Class
• Anticonvulsant, antineuralgic for chronic pain, alpha 2 delta ligand at voltage-sensitive calcium channels

Commonly Prescribed For
(bold for FDA approved)
• **Diabetic peripheral neuropathy**
• **Postherpetic neuralgia**
• Peripheral neuropathic pain
• Partial seizures with or without secondary generalization (adjunctive)
• Generalized anxiety disorder
• Panic disorder
• Social anxiety disorder
• Fibromyalgia

 How The Drug Works
• Is a leucine analogue and is transported both into the blood from the gut and also across the blood-brain barrier into the brain from the blood by the system L transport system (a sodium independent transporter) as well as by additional sodium-dependent amino acid transporter systems
✳ Binds to the alpha 2 delta subunit of voltage-sensitive calcium channels
• This closes N and P/Q presynaptic calcium channels, diminishing excessive neuronal activity and neurotransmitter release
• Although structurally related to gamma-aminobutyric acid (GABA), no known direct actions on GABA or its receptors

How Long Until It Works
• Can reduce neuropathic pain and anxiety within a week
• Should reduce seizures by 2 weeks
• If it is not producing clinical benefits within 6–8 weeks, it may require a dosage increase or it may not work at all

If It Works
• The goal of treatment of neuropathic pain, seizures, and anxiety disorders is to reduce symptoms as much as possible, and if necessary in combination with other treatments
• Treatment of neuropathic pain most often reduces but does not eliminate all symptoms and is not a cure since symptoms usually recur after medicine stopped
• Continue treatment until all symptoms are gone or until improvement is stable and then continue treating indefinitely as long as improvement persists

If It Doesn't Work (for neuropathic pain)
• Many patients only have a partial response where some symptoms are improved but others persist
• Other patients may be nonresponders, sometimes called treatment-resistant or treatment-refractory
• Consider increasing dose, switching to another agent or adding an appropriate augmenting agent
• Consider biofeedback or hypnosis for pain
• Consider psychotherapy for anxiety
• Consider the presence of noncompliance and counsel patient
• Consider evaluation for another diagnosis or for a comorbid condition (e.g., medical illness, substance abuse, etc.)

 Best Augmenting Combos for Partial Response or Treatment-Resistance
✳ In addition to being a first-line treatment for neuropathic pain and anxiety disorders, pregabalin is itself an augmenting agent to numerous other anticonvulsants in treating epilepsy
• For postherpetic neuralgia, pregabalin can decrease concomitant opiate use
✳ For neuropathic pain, tricyclic antidepressants and SNRIs as well as tiagabine, other anticonvulsants, and even opiates can augment pregabalin if done by experts while carefully monitoring in difficult cases
• For anxiety, SSRIs, SNRIs, or benzodiazepines can augment pregabalin

Tests
• None for healthy individuals

SIDE EFFECTS

How Drug Causes Side Effects
- CNS side effects may be due to excessive blockade of voltage-sensitive calcium channels

Notable Side Effects
* Sedation, dizziness
- Ataxia, fatigue, tremor, dysarthria, paraesthesia, memory impairment, coordination abnormal, impaired attention, confusion, euphoric mood, irritability
- Vomiting, dry mouth, constipation, weight gain, increased appetite, flatulence
- Blurred vision, diplopia
- Peripheral edema
- Libido decreased, erectile dysfunction

 Life Threatening or Dangerous Side Effects
- None

Weight Gain

- Occurs in significant minority

Sedation

- Many experience and/or can be significant in amount
- Dose-related
- Can wear off with time

What To Do About Side Effects
- Wait
- Wait
- Wait
- Take more of the dose at night to reduce daytime sedation
- Lower the dose
- Switch to another agent

Best Augmenting Agents for Side Effects
- Many side effects cannot be improved with an augmenting agent

DOSING AND USE

Usual Dosage Range
- 150–600 mg/day in 2–3 doses

Dosage Forms
- Capsule 25 mg, 50 mg, 75 mg, 100 mg, 150 mg, 200 mg, 300 mg

How to Dose
- Neuropathic pain: initial 150 mg/day in 2–3 doses; can increase to 300 mg/day in 2–3 doses after 3–7 days; can increase to 600 mg/day in 2–3 doses after 7 more days; maximum dose generally 600 mg/day
- Seizures: initial 150 mg/day in 2–3 doses; can increase to 300 mg/day in 2–3 doses after 7 days; can increase to 600 mg/day in 2–3 doses after 7 more days; maximum dose generally 600 mg/day

 Dosing Tips
* Generally given in one-third to one-sixth the dose of gabapentin
- If pregabalin is added to a second sedating agent, such as another anticonvulsant, a benzodiazepine, or an opiate, the titration period should be at least a week to improve tolerance to sedation
- Most patients only need to take pregabalin twice daily
- At the high end of the dosing range, tolerability may be enhanced by splitting dose into 3 or more divided doses
- For intolerable sedation, can give most of the dose at night and less during the day
- To improve slow-wave sleep, may only need to take pregabalin at bedtime
- May be taken with or without food

Overdose
- No fatalities

Long-Term Use
- Safe

Habit Forming
- No

How to Stop
- Taper over a minimum of 1 week
- Epilepsy patients may seize upon withdrawal, especially if withdrawal is abrupt

• Discontinuation symptoms uncommon

Pharmacokinetics
• Pregabalin is not metabolized but excreted intact renally
• Elimination half-life approximately 5–7 hours

 Drug Interactions
• Pregabalin has not been shown to have significant pharmacokinetic drug interactions
• Because pregabalin is excreted unchanged, it is unlikely to have significant pharmacokinetic drug interactions
• May add to or potentiate the sedative effects of oxycodone, lorazepam, and alcohol

 Other Warnings/ Precautions
• Dizziness and sedation could increase the chances of accidental injury (falls) in the elderly
• Increased incidence of hemangiosarcoma at high doses in mice involves platelet changes and associated endothelial cell proliferation not present in rats or humans; no evidence to suggest an associated risk for humans

Do Not Use
• If there is a proven allergy to pregabalin or gabapentin
• If patient has a problem of galactose intolerance, the Lapp lactase deficiency, or glucose-galactose malabsorption

SPECIAL POPULATIONS

Renal Impairment
• Pregabalin is renally excreted, so the dose may need to be lowered
• Dosing can be adjusted according to creatinine clearance, such that patients with clearance below 15 mL/min should receive 25–75 mg/day in 1 dose, patients with clearance between 15–29 mL/min should receive 25–150 mg/day in 1–2 doses, and patients with clearance between 30–59 mL/min should receive 75–300 mg/day in 2–3 doses

• Starting dose should be at the bottom of the range; titrate as usual up to maximum dose
• Can be removed by hemodialysis; patients receiving hemodialysis may require a supplemental dose of pregabalin following hemodialysis (25–100 mg)

Hepatic Impairment
• Dose adjustment not necessary

Cardiac Impairment
• No specific recommendations

Elderly
• Some patients may tolerate lower doses better
• Elderly patients may be more susceptible to adverse effects

 Children and Adolescents
• Safety and efficacy have not been established
• Use should be reserved for the expert

 Pregnancy
• Some animal studies have shown adverse effects, no controlled studies in humans
• Use in women of childbearing potential requires weighing potential benefits to the mother against the risks to the fetus
• Antiepileptic Drug Pregnancy Registry: (888) 233-2334
• Taper drug if discontinuing
• Seizures, even mild seizures, may cause harm to the embryo/fetus

Breast Feeding
• Unknown if pregabalin is secreted in human breast milk, but all psychotropics assumed to be secreted in breast milk
✳ Recommended either to discontinue drug or bottle feed
• If drug is continued while breast feeding, infant should be monitored for possible adverse effects
• If infant becomes irritable or sedated, breast feeding or drug may need to be discontinued

PREGABALIN (continued)

THE ART OF PSYCHOPHARMACOLOGY

Potential Advantages
- First-line for diabetic peripheral neuropathy
- Fibromyalgia
- Anxiety disorders
- Sleep
- Has relatively mild side effect profile
- Has few pharmacokinetic drug interactions
- More potent and probably better tolerated than gabapentin

Potential Disadvantages
- Requires 2–3 times a day dosing
- Not yet approved for anxiety disorders
- Not yet available in the United States

Primary Target Symptoms
- Seizures
- Pain
- Anxiety

 Pearls

✳ One of the first treatments approved for neuropathic pain associated with diabetic peripheral neuropathy
- Also approved in postherpetic neuralgia
- Improves sleep disruption as well as pain in patients with painful diabetic peripheral neuropathy or postherpetic neuralgia
- Improves pain and sleep disruption associated with fibromyalgia

- Well-studied in epilepsy, peripheral neuropathic pain, and generalized anxiety disorder
✳ Off-label use for generalized anxiety disorder, panic disorder, and social anxiety disorder may be justified
- May have uniquely robust therapeutic actions for both the somatic and the psychic symptoms of generalized anxiety disorder
✳ Off-label use as an adjunct for bipolar disorder may not be justified
✳ One of the few agents that enhances slow-wave delta sleep, which may be helpful in chronic neuropathic pain syndromes
- Pregabalin is generally well-tolerated, with only mild adverse effects
✳ Although no head-to-head studies, appears to be better tolerated and more consistently efficacious at high doses than gabapentin
✳ Drug absorption and clinical efficacy may be more consistent at high doses for pregabalin compared to gabapentin because of the higher potency of pregabalin and the fact that, unlike gabapentin, it is transported by more than one transport system

 Suggested Reading

Hovinga CA. Novel anticonvulsant medications in development. Expert Opin Investig Drugs 2002;11:1387–406.

Lauria-Horner BA, Pohl RB. Pregabalin: a new anxiolytic. Expert Opin Investig Drugs 2003; 12:663–72.

Stahl SM. Anticonvulsants and the relief of chronic pain: pregabalin and gabapentin as alpha(2)delta ligands at voltage-gated calcium channels. J Clin Psychiatry 2004;65:596–7.

Stahl SM. Anticonvulsants as anxiolytics, part 2: Pregabalin and gabapentin as alpha(2)delta ligands at voltage-gated calcium channels. J Clin Psychiatry 2004;65:460–1.

QUETIAPINE

Brands • Seroquel
see index for additional brand names

Generic? Not in U.S., Europe, or Japan

 Class

• Atypical antipsychotic (serotonin-dopamine antagonist; second generation antipsychotic; also a mood stabilizer)

Commonly Prescribed For
(bold for FDA approved)
• **Schizophrenia**
• **Acute mania (monotherapy and adjunct to lithium or valproate)**
• Other psychotic disorders
• Bipolar maintenance
• Bipolar depression
• Mixed mania
• Behavioral disturbances in dementias
• Behavioral disturbances in Parkinson's disease and Lewy Body dementia
• Psychosis associated with levodopa treatment in Parkinson's disease
• Behavioral disturbances in children and adolescents
• Disorders associated with problems with impulse control
• Severe treatment-resistant anxiety

 How The Drug Works

• Blocks dopamine 2 receptors, reducing positive symptoms of psychosis and stabilizing affective symptoms
• Blocks serotonin 2A receptors, causing enhancement of dopamine release in certain brain regions and thus reducing motor side effects and possibly improving cognitive and affective symptoms
• Interactions at a myriad of other neurotransmitter receptors may contribute to quetiapine's efficacy
✱ Specifically, actions at 5HT1A receptors may contribute to efficacy for cognitive and affective symptoms in some patients, especially at moderate to high doses

How Long Until It Works

• Psychotic and manic symptoms can improve within 1 week, but it may take several weeks for full effect on behavior as well as on cognition and affective stabilization
• Classically recommended to wait at least 4–6 weeks to determine efficacy of drug, but in practice some patients require up to 16–20 weeks to show a good response, especially on cognitive symptoms

If It Works

• Most often reduces positive symptoms in schizophrenia but does not eliminate them
• Can improve negative symptoms, as well as aggressive, cognitive, and affective symptoms in schizophrenia
• Most schizophrenic patients do not have a total remission of symptoms but rather a reduction of symptoms by about a third
• Perhaps 5–15% of schizophrenic patients can experience an overall improvement of greater than 50–60%, especially when receiving stable treatment for more than a year
• Such patients are considered super-responders or "awakeners" since they may be well enough to be employed, live independently, and sustain long-term relationships
• Many bipolar patients may experience a reduction of symptoms by half or more
• Continue treatment until reaching a plateau of improvement
• After reaching a satisfactory plateau, continue treatment for at least a year after first episode of psychosis
• For second and subsequent episodes of psychosis, treatment may need to be indefinite
• Even for first episodes of psychosis, it may be preferable to continue treatment indefinitely to avoid subsequent episodes
• Treatment may not only reduce mania but also prevent recurrences of mania in bipolar disorder

If It Doesn't Work

• Try one of the other atypical antipsychotics (risperidone, olanzapine, ziprasidone, aripiprazole, amisulpride)
• If 2 or more antipsychotic monotherapies do not work, consider clozapine
• If no first-line atypical antipsychotic is effective, consider higher doses or augmentation with valproate or lamotrigine
• Some patients may require treatment with a conventional antipsychotic

- Consider noncompliance and switch to another antipsychotic with fewer side effects or to an antipsychotic that can be given by depot injection
- Consider initiating rehabilitation and psychotherapy
- Consider presence of concomitant drug abuse

Best Augmenting Combos for Partial Response or Treatment-Resistance

- Valproic acid (valproate, divalproex, divalproex ER)
- Other mood stabilizing anticonvulsants (carbamazepine, oxcarbazepine, lamotrigine)
- Lithium
- Benzodiazepines

Tests

Before starting an atypical antipsychotic

✳ Weigh all patients and track BMI during treatment
- Get baseline personal and family history of diabetes, obesity, dyslipidemia, hypertension, and cardiovascular disease
✳ Get waist circumference (at umbilicus), blood pressure, fasting plasma glucose, and fasting lipid profile
- Determine if the patient is
  - overweight (BMI 25.0–29.9)
  - obese (BMI ≥30)
  - has pre-diabetes (fasting plasma glucose 100–125 mg/dl)
  - has diabetes (fasting plasma glucose >126 mg/dl)
  - has hypertension (BP >140/90 mm Hg)
  - has dyslipidemia (increased total cholesterol, LDL cholesterol, and triglycerides; decreased HDL cholesterol)
- Treat or refer such patients for treatment, including nutrition and weight management, physical activity counseling, smoking cessation, and medical management

Monitoring after starting an atypical antipsychotic

✳ BMI monthly for 3 months, then quarterly
✳ Blood pressure, fasting plasma glucose, fasting lipids within 3 months and then annually, but earlier and more frequently for patients with diabetes or who have gained >5% of initial weight

- Treat or refer for treatment and consider switching to another atypical antipsychotic for patients who become overweight, obese, pre-diabetic, diabetic, hypertensive, or dyslipidemic while receiving an atypical antipsychotic
✳ Even in patients without known diabetes, be vigilant for the rare but life threatening onset of diabetic ketoacidosis, which always requires immediate treatment, by monitoring for the rapid onset of polyuria, polydipsia, weight loss, nausea, vomiting, dehydration, rapid respiration, weakness and clouding of sensorium, even coma
- Although U.S. manufacturer recommends 6-month eye checks for cataracts, clinical experience suggests this may be unnecessary

SIDE EFFECTS

How Drug Causes Side Effects

- By blocking histamine 1 receptors in the brain, it can cause sedation and possibly weight gain
- By blocking alpha 1 adrenergic receptors, it can cause dizziness, sedation, and hypotension
- By blocking muscarinic 1 receptors, it can cause dry mouth, constipation, and sedation
- By blocking dopamine 2 receptors in the striatum, it can cause motor side effects (rare)
- Mechanism of weight gain and increased incidence of diabetes and dyslipidemia with atypical antipsychotics is unknown

Notable Side Effects

✳ May increase risk for diabetes and dyslipidemia
✳ Dizziness, sedation
- Dry mouth, constipation, dyspepsia, abdominal pain, weight gain
- Tachycardia
- Orthostatic hypotension, usually during initial dose titration
- Theoretical risk of tardive dyskinesia

Life Threatening or Dangerous Side Effects

- Hyperglycemia, in some cases extreme and associated with ketoacidosis or

hyperosmolar coma or death, has been reported in patients taking atypical antipsychotics
- Rare neuroleptic malignant syndrome (much reduced risk compared to conventional antipsychotics)
- Rare seizures
- Increased risk of death and cerebrovascular events in elderly patients with dementia-related psychosis

Weight Gain

unusual   not unusual   **common**   problematic

- Many patients experience and/or can be significant in amount at effective antipsychotic doses
- Can become a health problem in some
- May be less than for some antipsychotics, more than for others

Sedation

unusual   not unusual   common   **problematic**

- Frequent and can be significant in amount
- Some patients may not tolerate it
- More than for some other antipsychotics, but never say always as not a problem in everyone
- Can wear off over time
- Can reemerge as dose increases and then wear off again over time
- Not necessarily increased as dose is raised

What To Do About Side Effects

- Wait
- Wait
- Wait
- Usually dosed twice daily, so take more of the total daily dose at bedtime to help reduce daytime sedation
- Start dosing low and increase slowly as side effects wear off at each dosing increment
- Weight loss, exercise programs, and medical management for high BMIs, diabetes, dyslipidemia
- Switch to another atypical antipsychotic

Best Augmenting Agents for Side Effects

- Many side effects cannot be improved with an augmenting agent

DOSING AND USE

Usual Dosage Range
- 150–750 mg/day (in 2 doses) for schizophrenia
- 400–800 mg/day (in 2 doses) for acute bipolar mania

Dosage Forms
- Tablets 25 mg, 100 mg, 200 mg, 300 mg

How to Dose
- (according to manufacturer for schizophrenia): initial 25 mg/day twice a day; increase by 25–50 mg twice a day each day until desired efficacy is reached; maximum approved dose 800 mg/day
- In practice, can start adults with schizophrenia under age 65 with same doses as recommended for acute bipolar mania
- (according to manufacturing for acute bipolar mania): initiate in twice daily doses, totaling 100 mg/day on day 1, increasing to 400 mg/day on day 4 in increments of up to 100 mg/day; further dosage adjustments up to 800 mg/day by day 6 should be in increments of no greater than 200 mg/day

 Dosing Tips

* **More may be much more:** Clinical practice suggests quetiapine often underdosed, then switched prior to adequate trials
- Clinical practice suggests that at low doses it may be a sedative hypnotic, possibly due to potent H1 antihistamine actions, but this is an expensive use for which there are many other options
* Initial target dose of 400–800 mg/day should be reached in most cases to optimize the chances of success in treating acute psychosis and acute mania, but many patients are not adequately dosed in clinical practice
- Many patients do well with a single daily oral dose, usually at bedtime
- May be lower cost than some other atypical antipsychotics at 200 mg twice daily, but higher doses can be among the most costly for atypical antipsychotics
- Recommended titration to 400 mg/day by the fourth day can often be achieved when necessary to control acute symptoms

- Rapid dose escalation in manic or psychotic patients may lesson sedative side effects
- ✱ Higher doses generally achieve greater response
- Rapid dose escalation in manic or psychotic patients may lesson sedative side effects
- ✱ Occasional patients may require more than 800–1000 mg/day
- Rather than raise the dose above these levels in acutely agitated patients requiring acute antipsychotic actions, consider augmentation with a benzodiazepine or conventional antipsychotic, either orally or intramuscularly
- Rather than raise the dose above these levels in partial responders, consider augmentation with a mood stabilizing anticonvulsant such as valproate or lamotrigine
- Children and elderly should generally be dosed at the lower end of the dosage spectrum

Overdose
- Rarely lethal in monotherapy overdose; sedation, slurred speech, hypotension

Long-Term Use
- Often used for long-term maintenance in schizophrenia, bipolar disorder, and various behavioral disorders

Habit Forming
- No

How to Stop
- Slow down-titration (over 6 to 8 weeks), especially when simultaneously beginning a new antipsychotic while switching (i.e., cross-titration)
- Rapid discontinuation may lead to rebound psychosis and worsening of symptoms

Pharmacokinetics
- Metabolites are inactive
- Parent drug has 6–7 hour half-life

 Drug Interactions
- CYP450 3A inhibitors and CYP450 2D6 inhibitors may reduce clearance of quetiapine and thus raise quetiapine

plasma levels, but dosage reduction of quetiapine usually not necessary
- May increase effect of anti-hypertensive agents

 Other Warnings/ Precautions
- In the U.S., manufacturer recommends examination for cataracts before and every 6 months after initiating quetiapine, but this does not seem to be necessary in clinical practice
- Quetiapine should be used cautiously in patients at risk for aspiration pneumonia, as dysphagia has been reported
- Priapism has been reported
- Use with caution in patients with known cardiovascular disease, cerebrovascular disease
- Use with caution in patients with conditions that predispose to hypotension (dehydration, overheating)

Do Not Use
- If there is a proven allergy to quetiapine

Renal Impairment
- No dose adjustment required

Hepatic Impairment
- Downward dose adjustment may be necessary

Cardiac Impairment
- Drug should be used with caution because of risk of orthostatic hypotension

Elderly
- Lower dose is generally used (e.g., 25–100 mg twice a day), although higher doses may be used if tolerated
- Although atypical antipsychotics are commonly used for behavioral disturbances in dementia, no agent has been approved for treatment of elderly patients with dementia-related psychosis
- Elderly patients with dementia-related psychosis treated with atypical antipsychotics are at an increased risk of death compared to placebo, and also have an increased risk of cerebrovascular events

Children and Adolescents

- Not officially recommended for patients under age 18
- Clinical experience and early data suggest quetiapine may be safe and effective for behavioral disturbances in children and adolescents
- Children and adolescents using quetiapine may need to be monitored more often than adults
- May tolerate lower doses better

 Pregnancy

- Risk Category C [some animal studies show adverse effects, no controlled studies in humans]
- Psychotic symptoms may worsen during pregnancy and some form of treatment may be necessary
- Quetiapine may be preferable to anticonvulsant mood stabilizers if treatment is required during pregnancy

Breast Feeding

- Unknown if quetiapine is secreted in human breast milk, but all psychotropics assumed to be secreted in breast milk
- Recommended either to discontinue drug or bottle feed
- Infants of women who choose to breast feed while on quetiapine should be monitored for possible adverse effects

THE ART OF PSYCHOPHARMACOLOGY

Potential Advantages

- Some cases of psychosis and bipolar disorder refractory to treatment with other antipsychotics
- ✳ Patients with Parkinson's disease who need an antipsychotic or mood stabilizer
- ✳ Patients with Lewy Body dementia who need an antipsychotic or mood stabilizer

Potential Disadvantages

- Patients requiring rapid onset of action
- Patients noncompliant with twice daily dosing
- Patients who have difficulty tolerating sedation

Primary Target Symptoms

- Positive symptoms of psychosis
- Negative symptoms of psychosis
- Cognitive symptoms
- Unstable mood (both depression and mania)
- Aggressive symptoms
- Insomnia and anxiety

 Pearls

- ✳ May be the preferred antipsychotic for psychosis in Parkinson's disease and Lewy Body dementia
- Anecdotal reports of efficacy in treatment-refractory cases and positive symptoms of psychoses other than schizophrenia
- ✳ Efficacy may be underestimated since quetiapine is often under-dosed in clinical practice
- ✳ Controlled data have demonstrated efficacy of quetiapine in bipolar depression
- More sedation than some other antipsychotics, which may be of benefit in acutely manic or psychotic patients but not for stabilized patients in long-term maintenance
- ✳ Essentially no motor side effects or prolactin elevation
- May have less weight gain than some antipsychotics, more than others
- ✳ Controversial as to whether quetiapine has more or less risk of diabetes and dyslipidemia than some other antipsychotics
- Can be a more expensive atypical antipsychotic than some others when dosed appropriately in schizophrenia or acute mania; some patients respond to moderate doses, which are less expensive
- Commonly used at low doses to augment other atypical antipsychotics, but such antipsychotic polypharmacy has not been systematically studied and can be quite expensive
- Anecdotal reports of efficacy in posttraumatic stress disorder, including symptoms of sleep disturbance and anxiety

Suggested Reading

Kapur S, Remington G. Atypical antipsychotics: new directions and new challenges in the treatment of schizophrenia. Annu Rev Med 2001;52:503–17.

Srisurapanont M, Disayavanish C, Taimkaew K. Quetiapine for schizophrenia. Cochrane Database Syst Rev 2000;3:CD000967.

Tandon R. Safety and tolerability: how do new generation "atypical" antipsychotics compare? Psychiatric Quarterly 2002;73:297–311.

Tandon R, Jibson MD. Efficacy of newer generation antipsychotics in the treatment of schizophrenia. Psychoneuroendocrinology 2003;28:9–26.

Yatham LN. Efficacy of atypical antipsychotics in mood disorders. J Clin Psychopharmacol 2003;23(3 Suppl 1):S9–14.

Brands • Risperdal • CONSTA
see index for additional brand names

Generic? Not in U.S. or Japan

Class

- Atypical antipsychotic (serotonin-dopamine antagonist; second generation antipsychotic; also a mood stabilizer)

Commonly Prescribed For
(bold for FDA approved)

- **Schizophrenia (oral, long-acting microspheres intramuscularly)**
- **Delaying relapse in schizophrenia (oral)**
- **Other psychotic disorders (oral)**
- **Acute mania/mixed mania (oral, monotherapy and adjunct to lithium or valproate)**
- Bipolar maintenance
- Bipolar depression
- Behavioral disturbances in dementias
- Behavioral disturbances in children and adolescents
- Disorders associated with problems with impulse control

How The Drug Works

- Blocks dopamine 2 receptors, reducing positive symptoms of psychosis and stabilizing affective symptoms
- Blocks serotonin 2A receptors, causing enhancement of dopamine release in certain brain regions and thus reducing motor side effects and possibly improving cognitive and affective symptoms
- Interactions at a myriad of other neurotransmitter receptors may contribute to risperidone's efficacy
- ✳ Specifically, alpha 2 antagonist properties may contribute to antidepressant actions

How Long Until It Works

- Psychotic and manic symptoms can improve within 1 week, but it may take several weeks for full effect on behavior as well as on cognition and affective stabilization
- Classically recommended to wait at least 4–6 weeks to determine efficacy of drug, but in practice some patients require up to 16–20 weeks to show a good response, especially on cognitive symptoms

If It Works

- Most often reduces positive symptoms in schizophrenia but does not eliminate them
- Can improve negative symptoms, as well as aggressive, cognitive, and affective symptoms in schizophrenia
- Most schizophrenic patients do not have a total remission of symptoms but rather a reduction of symptoms by about a third
- Perhaps 5–15% of schizophrenic patients can experience an overall improvement of greater than 50–60%, especially when receiving stable treatment for more than a year
- Such patients are considered super-responders or "awakeners" since they may be well enough to be employed, live independently, and sustain long-term relationships
- Many bipolar patients may experience a reduction of symptoms by half or more
- Continue treatment until reaching a plateau of improvement
- After reaching a satisfactory plateau, continue treatment for at least a year after first episode of psychosis
- For second and subsequent episodes of psychosis, treatment may need to be indefinite
- Even for first episodes of psychosis, it may be preferable to continue treatment indefinitely to avoid subsequent episodes
- Treatment may not only reduce mania but also prevent recurrences of mania in bipolar disorder

If It Doesn't Work

- Try one of the other atypical antipsychotics (olanzapine, quetiapine, ziprasidone, aripiprazole, amisulpride)
- If 2 or more antipsychotic monotherapies do not work, consider clozapine
- If no first-line atypical antipsychotic is effective, consider higher doses or augmentation with valproate or lamotrigine
- Some patients may require treatment with a conventional antipsychotic
- Consider noncompliance and switch to another antipsychotic with fewer side effects or to an antipsychotic that can be given by depot injection

- Consider initiating rehabilitation and psychotherapy
- Consider presence of concomitant drug abuse

Best Augmenting Combos for Partial Response or Treatment-Resistance

- Valproic acid (valproate, divalproex, divalproex ER)
- Other mood stabilizing anticonvulsants (carbamazepine, oxcarbazepine, lamotrigine)
- Lithium
- Benzodiazepines

Tests

Before starting an atypical antipsychotic

✽ Weigh all patients and track BMI during treatment
- Get baseline personal and family history of diabetes, obesity, dyslipidemia, hypertension, and cardiovascular disease

✽ Get waist circumference (at umbilicus), blood pressure, fasting plasma glucose, and fasting lipid profile
- Determine if the patient is
  - overweight (BMI 25.0–29.9)
  - obese (BMI ≥30)
  - has pre-diabetes (fasting plasma glucose 100–125 mg/dl)
  - has diabetes (fasting plasma glucose >126 mg/dl)
  - has hypertension (BP >140/90 mm Hg)
  - has dyslipidemia (increased total cholesterol, LDL cholesterol, and triglycerides; decreased HDL cholesterol)
- Treat or refer such patients for treatment, including nutrition and weight management, physical activity counseling, smoking cessation, and medical management

Monitoring after starting an atypical antipsychotic

✽ BMI monthly for 3 months, then quarterly

✽ Blood pressure, fasting plasma glucose, fasting lipids within 3 months and then annually, but earlier and more frequently for patients with diabetes or who have gained >5% of initial weight
- Treat or refer for treatment and consider switching to another atypical antipsychotic for patients who become overweight, obese, pre-diabetic, diabetic, hypertensive, or dyslipidemic while receiving an atypical antipsychotic

✽ Even in patients without known diabetes, be vigilant for the rare but life threatening onset of diabetic ketoacidosis, which always requires immediate treatment, by monitoring for the rapid onset of polyuria, polydipsia, weight loss, nausea, vomiting, dehydration, rapid respiration, weakness and clouding of sensorium, even coma
- Should check blood pressure in the elderly before starting and for the first few weeks of treatment
- Monitoring elevated prolactin levels of dubious clinical benefit

SIDE EFFECTS

How Drug Causes Side Effects

- By blocking alpha 1 adrenergic receptors, it can cause dizziness, sedation, and hypotension
- By blocking dopamine 2 receptors in the striatum, it can cause motor side effects, especially at high doses
- By blocking dopamine 2 receptors in the pituitary, it can cause elevations in prolactin
- Mechanism of weight gain and increased incidence of diabetes and dyslipidemia with atypical antipsychotics is unknown

Notable Side Effects

✽ May increase risk for diabetes and dyslipidemia

✽ Dose-dependent extrapyramidal symptoms

✽ Dose-related hyperprolactinemia
- Rare tardive dyskinesia (much reduced risk compared to conventional antipsychotics)
- Dizziness, insomnia, headache, anxiety, sedation
- Nausea, constipation, abdominal pain, weight gain
- Rare orthostatic hypotension, usually during initial dose titration
- Tachycardia, sexual dysfunction

Life Threatening or Dangerous Side Effects

- Hyperglycemia, in some cases extreme and associated with ketoacidosis or hyperosmolar coma or death, has been reported in patients taking atypical antipsychotics

- Increased risk of death and cerebrovascular events in elderly patients with dementia-related psychosis
- Rare neuroleptic malignant syndrome (much reduced risk compared to conventional antipsychotics)
- Rare seizures

Weight Gain

unusual — not unusual — common — problematic

- Many patients experience and/or can be significant in amount
- Can become a health problem in some
- May be less than for some antipsychotics, more than for others

Sedation

unusual — not unusual — common — problematic

- Many patients experience and/or can be significant in amount
- Usually transient
- May be less than for some antipsychotics, more than for others

What To Do About Side Effects

- Wait
- Wait
- Wait
- Take at bedtime to help reduce daytime sedation
- Anticholinergics may reduce motor side effects when present
- Weight loss, exercise programs, and medical management for high BMIs, diabetes, dyslipidemia
- Switch to another atypical antipsychotic

Best Augmenting Agents for Side Effects

- Benztropine or trihexyphenidyl for motor side effects
- Many side effects cannot be improved with an augmenting agent

DOSING AND USE

Usual Dosage Range

- 2–8 mg/day orally for acute psychosis and bipolar disorder
- 0.5–2.0 mg/day orally for children and elderly

- 25–50 mg depot intramuscularly every 2 weeks

Dosage Forms

- Tablets 0.25 mg, 0.5 mg, 1 mg, 2 mg, 3 mg, 4 mg, 6 mg
- Orally disintegrating tablets 0.5 mg, 1 mg, 2 mg
- Liquid 1 mg/mL — 30 mL bottle
- Risperidone long-acting depot microspheres formulation for deep intramuscular administration 25 mg vial/kit, 37.5 mg vial/kit, 50 mg vial/kit

How to Dose

- In adults with psychosis in non-emergent settings, initial dosage recommendation is 1 mg/day orally in 2 divided doses
- Increase each day by 1 mg/day orally until desired efficacy is reached
- Maximum generally 16 mg/day orally
- Typically maximum effect is seen at 4–8 mg/day orally
- Can be administered on a once daily schedule as well as twice daily orally
- Long-acting risperidone is not recommended for patients who have not first demonstrated tolerability to oral risperidone
- Long-acting risperidone should be administered every 2 weeks by deep intramuscular gluteal injection
- Oral antipsychotic medication should be given with the first injection of long-acting risperidone and continued for 3 weeks, then discontinued
- Long-acting risperidone should only be administered by a health care professional
- Typically maximum effect with long-acting risperidone is seen at 25–50 mg every 2 weeks; maximum recommended dose is 50 mg every 2 weeks
- Titration of long-acting risperidone should occur at intervals of no less than 4 weeks
- Two different dosage strengths of long-acting risperidone should not be combined in a single administration

 Dosing Tips – Oral Formulation

* **Less may be more:** lowering the dose in some patients with stable efficacy but side effects may reduce side effects without loss of efficacy, especially for doses over 6 mg/day orally

✳ Target doses for best efficacy/best tolerability in many adults with psychosis or bipolar disorder may be 2–6 mg/day (average 4.5 mg/day) orally
- Patients who respond to these doses may have one of the lowest drug costs among the atypical antipsychotics
- Low doses may not be adequate in difficult patients
- Rather than raise the dose above these levels in acutely agitated patients requiring acute antipsychotic actions, consider augmentation with a benzodiazepine or conventional antipsychotic, either orally or intramuscularly
- Rather than raise the dose above these levels in partial responders, consider augmentation with a mood stabilizing anticonvulsant, such as valproate or lamotrigine
- Approved for use up to 16 mg/day orally, but data suggest that risk of extrapyramidal symptoms is increased above 6 mg/day
- Risperidone oral solution is not compatible with cola or tea
- Children and elderly may need to have oral twice daily dosing during initiation and titration of drug dosing and then can switch to oral once daily when maintenance dose is reached
- Children and elderly should generally be dosed at the lower end of the dosage spectrum

Dosing Tips – Long-Acting Microsphere Depot Formulation

✳ When initiating long-acting risperidone formulation by intramuscular injection, onset of action can be delayed for 2 weeks while microspheres are being absorbed
✳ For antipsychotic coverage during initiation of long-acting risperidone, continue ongoing treatment with an oral antipsychotic or initiate treatment with some oral antipsychotic for 3 weeks
- Steady-state plasma concentrations are reached after 4 injections of long-acting risperidone and maintained for 4–6 weeks after the last injection
- For missed long-acting risperidone injections 2 or more weeks late (i.e., 28 or more days following last injection), may need to provide antipsychotic coverage

with oral administration for 3 weeks while reinitiating injections
- For missed long-acting risperidone injections up to 2 weeks late (i.e., within 28 days of last injection), may not need to provide oral coverage
- Long-acting risperidone must be kept refrigerated
- Must deliver each syringe in full since drug is not in a solution (i.e., half a syringe is not necessarily half the drug dose)

Overdose
- Rarely lethal in monotherapy overdose; sedation, rapid heartbeat, convulsions, low blood pressure, difficulty breathing

Long-Term Use
- Approved to delay relapse in long-term treatment of schizophrenia
- Often used for long-term maintenance in bipolar disorder and various behavioral disorders

Habit Forming
- No

How to Stop
- Slow down-titration of oral formulation (over 6 to 8 weeks), especially when simultaneously beginning a new antipsychotic while switching (i.e., cross-titration)
- Rapid oral discontinuation may lead to rebound psychosis and worsening of symptoms

Pharmacokinetics
- Metabolites are active
- Metabolized by CYP450 2D6
- Parent drug of oral formulation has 20–24 hour half-life
- Long-acting risperidone has 3–6 day half-life
- Long-acting risperidone has elimination phase of approximately 7–8 weeks after last injection

Drug Interactions
- May increase effect of anti-hypertensive agents
- May antagonize levodopa, dopamine agonists
- Clearance of risperidone may be reduced and thus plasma levels increased by

clozapine; dosing adjustment usually not necessary
- Co-administration with carbamazepine may decrease plasma levels of risperidone
- Co-administration with fluoxetine and paroxetine may increase plasma levels of risperidone
- Since risperidone is metabolized by CYP450 2D6, any agent that inhibits this enzyme could theoretically raise risperidone plasma levels; however, dose reduction of risperidone is usually not necessary when such combinations are used

 Other Warnings/ Precautions

- Use with caution in patients with conditions that predispose to hypotension (dehydration, overheating)
- Risperidone should be used cautiously in patients at risk for aspiration pneumonia, as dysphagia has been reported
- Priapism has been reported

Do Not Use
- If there is a proven allergy to risperidone

SPECIAL POPULATIONS

Renal Impairment
- Initial 0.5 mg orally twice a day for first week; increase to 1 mg twice a day during second week
- Long-acting risperidone should not be administered unless patient has demonstrated tolerability of at least 2 mg/day orally
- Long-acting risperidone should be dosed at 25 mg every 2 weeks; oral administration should be continued for 3 weeks after the first injection

Hepatic Impairment
- Initial 0.5 mg orally twice a day for first week; increase to 1 mg twice a day during second week
- Long-acting risperidone should not be administered unless patient has demonstrated tolerability of at least 2 mg/day orally
- Long-acting risperidone should be dosed at 25 mg every two weeks; oral

administration should be continued for 3 weeks after the first injection

Cardiac Impairment
- Drug should be used with caution because of risk of orthostatic hypotension
- ✳ When administered to elderly patients with atrial fibrillation, may increase the chances of stroke

Elderly
- Initial 0.5 mg orally twice a day; increase by 0.5 mg twice a day; titrate once a week for doses above 1.5 mg twice a day
- Recommended dose of long-acting risperidone is 25 mg every 2 weeks; oral administration should be continued for 3 weeks after the first injection
- Although atypical antipsychotics are commonly used for behavioral disturbances in dementia, no agent has been approved for treatment of elderly patients with dementia-related psychosis
- Elderly patients with dementia-related psychosis treated with atypical antipsychotics are at an increased risk of death compared to placebo, and also have an increased risk of cerebrovascular events

 Children and Adolescents

- Safety and effectiveness have not been established
- ✳ However, risperidone is the most frequently used atypical antipsychotic in children and adolescents
- Clinical experience and early data suggest risperidone is safe and effective for behavioral disturbances in children and adolescents
- Risperidone received a not approvable letter from the FDA for the treatment of autism
- Children and adolescents using risperidone may need to be monitored more often than adults

 Pregnancy
- Risk Category C [some animal studies show adverse effects, no controlled studies in humans]

- Psychotic symptoms may worsen during pregnancy and some form of treatment may be necessary
- Early findings of infants exposed to risperidone in utero do not show adverse consequences
- Risperidone may be preferable to anticonvulsant mood stabilizers if treatment is required during pregnancy
- Effects of hyperprolactinemia on the fetus are unknown

Breast Feeding

- Unknown if risperidone is secreted in human breast milk, but all psychotropics assumed to be secreted in breast milk
- ✳ Recommended either to discontinue drug or bottle feed
- Infants of women who choose to breast feed while on risperidone should be monitored for possible adverse effects

THE ART OF PSYCHOPHARMACOLOGY

Potential Advantages

- Some cases of psychosis and bipolar disorder refractory to treatment with other antipsychotics
- ✳ Often a preferred treatment for dementia with aggressive features
- ✳ Often a preferred atypical antipsychotic for children with behavioral disturbances of multiple causations
- ✳ Non-compliant patients (long-acting risperidone)
- ✳ Long-term outcomes may be enhanced when compliance is enhanced (long-acting risperidone)

Potential Disadvantages

- Patients for whom elevated prolactin may not be desired (e.g., possibly pregnant patients; pubescent girls with amenorrhea; postmenopausal women with low estrogen who do not take estrogen replacement therapy)

Primary Target Symptoms

- Positive symptoms of psychosis

- Negative symptoms of psychosis
- Cognitive functioning
- Unstable mood (both depression and mania)
- Aggressive symptoms

 Pearls

- ✳ Well accepted for treatment of agitation and aggression in elderly demented patients
- ✳ Well accepted for treatment of behavioral symptoms in children and adolescents, but may have more sedation and weight gain in pediatric populations than in adult populations
- Risperidone received a not approvable letter for treatment of autism
- Many anecdotal reports of utility in treatment-refractory cases and for positive symptoms of psychosis in disorders other than schizophrenia
- Only atypical antipsychotic to consistently raise prolactin, but this is of unproven and uncertain clinical significance
- Hyperprolactinemia in women with low estrogen may accelerate osteoporosis
- Less weight gain than some antipsychotics, more than others
- Less sedation than some antipsychotics, more than others
- Risperidone is one of the least expensive atypical antipsychotics within the usual therapeutic dosing range
- Increased risk of stroke may be most relevant in the elderly with atrial fibrillation
- ✳ Controversial as to whether risperidone has more or less risk of diabetes and dyslipidemia than some other antipsychotics
- May cause more motor side effects than some other atypical antipsychotics, especially when administered to patients with Parkinson's disease or Lewy Body dementia
- ✳ Only atypical antipsychotic with a long-acting depot formulation

Suggested Reading

Kapur S, Remington G. Atypical antipsychotics: new directions and new challenges in the treatment of schizophrenia. Annu Rev Med 2001;52:503–17.

Schweitzer I. Does risperidone have a place in the treatment of nonschizophrenic patients? International Clinical Psychopharmacology 2001;16:1–19.

Tandon R. Safety and tolerability: how do new generation "atypical" antipsychotics compare? Psychiatric Quarterly 2002;73:297–311.

Tandon R, Jibson MD. Efficacy of newer generation antipsychotics in the treatment of schizophrenia. Psychoneuroendocrinology 2003;28:9–26.

Yatham LN. Efficacy of atypical antipsychotics in mood disorders. J Clin Psychopharmacol 2003;23(3 Suppl 1):S9–14.

TOPIRAMATE

THERAPEUTICS

Brands
- Topamax
- Epitomax
- Topamac
- Topimax

see index for additional brand names

Generic? No

Class
- Anticonvulsant, voltage-sensitive sodium channel modulator

Commonly Prescribed For
(bold for FDA approved)
- **Partial onset seizures (adjunctive; adults and pediatric patients 2–16 years of age)**
- **Primary generalized tonic-clonic seizures (adjunctive; adults and pediatric patients 2–16 years of age)**
- **Seizures associated with Lennox-Gastaut Syndrome (2 years of age or older)**
- **Migraine prophylaxis**
- Bipolar disorder (adjunctive; no longer in development)
- Psychotropic drug-induced weight gain
- Binge-eating disorder

How The Drug Works
* Blocks voltage-sensitive sodium channels by an unknown mechanism
- Inhibits release of glutamate
- Potentiates activity of gamma-aminobutyric acid (GABA)
- Carbonic anhydrase inhibitor

How Long Until It Works
- Should reduce seizures by 2 weeks
- Not clear that it has mood stabilizing properties, but some bipolar patients may respond and if so, it may take several weeks to months to optimize an effect on mood stabilization

If It Works
- The goal of treatment is complete remission of symptoms (e.g., mania, seizures, migraine)
- Continue treatment until all symptoms are gone or until improvement is stable and then continue treating indefinitely as long as improvement persists

- Continue treatment indefinitely to avoid recurrence of mania, seizures, and headaches

If It Doesn't Work (for bipolar disorder)
* May only be effective in a subset of bipolar patients, in some patients who fail to respond to other mood stabilizers, or it may not work at all
* Consider increasing dose or switching to another agent with better demonstrated efficacy in bipolar disorder

 Best Augmenting Combos for Partial Response or Treatment-Resistance
- Topiramate is itself a second-line augmenting agent for numerous other anticonvulsants, lithium, and antipsychotics in treating bipolar disorder

Tests
* Baseline and periodic serum bicarbonate levels to monitor for hyperchloremic, non-anion gap metabolic acidosis (i.e., decreased serum bicarbonate below the normal reference range in the absence of chronic respiratory alkalosis)

SIDE EFFECTS

How Drug Causes Side Effects
- CNS side effects theoretically due to excessive actions at voltage-sensitive sodium channels
- Weak inhibition of carbonic anhydrase may lead to kidney stones and paresthesias
- Inhibition of carbonic anhydrase may also lead to metabolic acidosis

Notable Side Effects
* Sedation, asthenia, dizziness, ataxia, parasthesia, nervousness, nystagmus, tremor
* Nausea, appetite loss, weight loss
- Blurred or double vision, mood problems, problems concentrating, confusion, memory problems, psychomotor retardation, language problems, speech problems, fatigue, taste perversion

Life Threatening or Dangerous Side Effects

✳ Metabolic acidosis
✳ Kidney stones
• Secondary narrow angle-closure glaucoma
• Oligohidrosis and hyperthermia (more common in children)
• Sudden unexplained deaths have occurred in epilepsy (unknown if related to topiramate use)

Weight Gain

unusual   not unusual   common   problematic

• Reported but not expected
✳ Patients may experience weight loss

Sedation

unusual   not unusual   common   problematic

• Many experience and/or can be significant in amount

What To Do About Side Effects

• Wait
• Wait
• Wait
• Take at night to reduce daytime sedation
• Increase fluid intake to reduce the risk of kidney stones
• Switch to another agent

Best Augmenting Agents for Side Effects

• Many side effects cannot be improved with an augmenting agent

---

DOSING AND USE

Usual Dosage Range

• Adults: 200–400 mg/day in 2 divided doses for epilepsy; 50–300 mg/day for adjunctive treatment of bipolar disorder

Dosage Forms

• Tablet 25 mg, 100 mg, 200 mg
• Sprinkle capsule 15 mg, 25 mg

How to Dose

• Adults: initial 25–50 mg/day; increase each week by 50 mg/day; administer in 2 divided doses; maximum dose generally 1600 mg/day
• Seizures (ages 2–16): see Children and Adolescents

 Dosing Tips

• Adverse effects may increase as dose increases
• Topiramate is available in a sprinkle capsule formulation, which can be swallowed whole or sprinkled over approximately a teaspoon of soft food (e.g., applesauce); the mixture should be consumed immediately
• Bipolar patients are generally administered doses at the lower end of the dosing range
• Slow upward titration from doses as low as 25 mg/day can reduce the incidence of unacceptable sedation
• Many bipolar patients do not tolerate more than 200 mg/day
✳ Weight loss is dose-related but most patients treated for weight gain receive doses at the lower end of the dosing range

Overdose

• No fatalities have been reported in monotherapy; convulsions, sedation, speech disturbance, blurred or double vision, metabolic acidosis, impaired coordination, hypotension, abdominal pain, agitation, dizziness

Long-Term Use

• Probably safe
• Periodic monitoring of serum bicarbonate levels may be required

Habit Forming

• No

How to Stop

• Taper
• Epilepsy patients may seize upon withdrawal, especially if withdrawal is abrupt
✳ Rapid discontinuation may increase the risk of relapse in bipolar patients
✳ Discontinuation symptoms uncommon

Pharmacokinetics

• Elimination half-life approximately 21 hours
• Renally excreted

Drug Interactions

- Carbamazepine, phenytoin, and valproate may increase the clearance of topiramate, and thus decrease topiramate levels, possibly requiring a higher dose of topiramate
- Topiramate may increase the clearance of phenytoin and thus decrease phenytoin levels, possibly requiring a higher dose of phenytoin
- Topiramate may increase the clearance of valproate and thus decrease valproate levels, possibly requiring a higher dose of valproate
- Topiramate may increase plasma levels of metformin; also, metformin may reduce clearance of topiramate and increase topiramate levels
- Topiramate may interact with carbonic anhydrase inhibitors to increase the risk of kidney stones
- Topiramate may reduce the effectiveness of oral contraceptives

⚠ **Other Warnings/ Precautions**

✳ If symptoms of metabolic acidosis develop (hyperventilation, fatigue, anorexia, cardiac arrhythmias, stupor), then dose may need to be reduced or treatment may need to be discontinued
- Depressive effects may be increased by other CNS depressants (alcohol, MAOIs, other anticonvulsants, etc.)
- Use with caution when combining with other drugs that predispose patients to heat-related disorders, including carbonic anhydrase inhibitors and anticholinergics

Do Not Use
- If there is a proven allergy to topiramate

SPECIAL POPULATIONS

Renal Impairment
- Topiramate is renally excreted, so the dose should be lowered by half
- Can be removed by hemodialysis; patients receiving hemodialysis may require supplemental doses of topiramate

Hepatic Impairment
- Drug should be used with caution

Cardiac Impairment
- Drug should be used with caution

Elderly
- Elderly patients may be more susceptible to adverse effects

 Children and Adolescents
- Approved for use in children age 2 and older for treatment of seizures
- Clearance is increased in pediatric patients
- Seizures (ages 2–16): initial 1–3 mg/kg/day at night; after 1 week increase by 1–3 mg/kg/day every 1–2 weeks with total daily dose administered in 2 divided doses; recommended dose generally 5–9 mg/kg/day in 2 divided doses

 Pregnancy
- Risk category C [some animal studies show adverse effects, no controlled studies in humans]
- Use in women of childbearing potential requires weighing potential benefits to the mother against the risks to the fetus
- Hypospadia has occurred in some male infants whose mothers took topiramate during pregnancy
✳ Lack of convincing efficacy for treatment of bipolar disorder suggests risk/benefit ratio is in favor of discontinuing topiramate in bipolar patients during pregnancy
✳ For bipolar patients, topiramate should generally be discontinued before anticipated pregnancies
- Antiepileptic Drug Pregnancy Registry: (888) 233-2334
- Taper drug if discontinuing
✳ For bipolar patients, given the risk of relapse in the postpartum period, mood stabilizer treatment, especially with agents with better evidence of efficacy than topiramate, should generally be restarted immediately after delivery if patient is unmedicated during pregnancy
✳ Atypical antipsychotics may be preferable to topiramate if treatment of bipolar disorder is required during pregnancy

- Bipolar symptoms may recur or worsen during pregnancy and some form of treatment may be necessary
- Seizures, even mild seizures, may cause harm to the embryo/fetus

Breast Feeding

- Some drug is found in mother's breast milk
- ✳ Recommended either to discontinue drug or bottle feed
- If drug is continued while breast feeding, infant should be monitored for possible adverse effects
- If infant shows signs of irritability or sedation, drug may need to be discontinued
- ✳ Bipolar disorder may recur during the postpartum period, particularly if there is a history of prior postpartum episodes of either depression or psychosis
- ✳ Relapse rates may be lower in women who receive prophylactic treatment for postpartum episodes of bipolar disorder
- Atypical antipsychotics and anticonvulsants such as valproate may be safer and more effective than topiramate during the postpartum period when treating nursing mother with bipolar disorder

THE ART OF PSYCHOPHARMACOLOGY

Potential Advantages

- Treatment-resistant bipolar disorder
- Patients who wish to avoid weight gain

Potential Disadvantages

- Efficacy in bipolar disorder uncertain
- Patients with a history of kidney stones or risks for metabolic acidosis

Primary Target Symptoms

- Incidence of seizures
- Unstable mood

Pearls

- Side effects may actually occur less often in pediatric patients
- Has been studied in a wide range of psychiatric disorders, including bipolar

disorder, posttraumatic stress disorder, binge-eating disorder, obesity and others
- Some anecdotes, case series, and open-label studies have been published and are widely known suggesting efficacy in bipolar disorder
- ✳ However, randomized clinical trials do not suggest efficacy in bipolar disorder; unfortunately these important studies have not been published by the manufacturer, who has dropped topiramate from further development as a mood stabilizer, though this is not widely known
- ✳ Misperceptions about topiramate's efficacy in bipolar disorder have led to its use in more patients than other agents with proven efficacy, such as lamotrigine
- ✳ Due to reported weight loss in some patients in trials with epilepsy, topiramate is commonly used to treat weight gain, especially in patients with psychotropic drug-induced weight gain
- ✳ Weight loss in epilepsy patients is dose related with more weight loss at high doses (mean 6.5 kg or 7.3% decline) and less weight loss at lower doses (mean 1.6 kg or 2.2% decline)
- ✳ Changes in weight were greatest in epilepsy patients who weighed the most at baseline (>100 kg), with mean loss of 9.6 kg or 8.4% decline, while those weighing <60 kg had only a mean loss of 1.3 kg or 2.5% decline
- ✳ Long-term studies demonstrate that weight losses in epilepsy patients were seen within the first 3 months of treatment and peaked at a mean of 6 kg after 12 to 18 months of treatment; however, weight tended to return to pretreatment levels after 18 months
- ✳ Some patients with psychotropic drug-induced weight gain may experience significant weight loss (>7% of body weight) with topiramate up to 200 mg/day for 3 months, but this is not typical, is not often sustained, and has not been systemically studied
- Early studies suggest potential efficacy in binge-eating disorder

Suggested Reading

Chengappa KR, Gershon S, Levine J. The evolving role of topiramate among other mood stabilizers in the management of bipolar disorder. Bipolar Disord. 2001; 3: 215–232.

Ormrod D, McClellan K. Topiramate: a review of its use in childhood epilepsy. Paediatr Drugs. 2001; 3: 293–319.

MacDonald KJ, Young LT. Newer antiepileptic drugs in bipolar disorder. CNS Drugs 2002;16:549–62.

Shank RP, Gardocki JF, Streeter AJ, Maryanoff BE. An overview of the preclinical aspects of topiramate: pharmacology, pharmacokinetics, and mechanism of action. Epilepsia. 2000; 41 (Suppl 1): S3–9.

Suppes T. Review of the use of topiramate for treatment of bipolar disorders. J Clin Psychopharmacol 2002;22:599–609.

VALPROATE

THERAPEUTICS

Brands
- Depakene
- Depacon
- Depakote, Depakote ER

see index for additional brand names

Generic? Yes (not for Depakote or Depakote ER)

 Class
- Anticonvulsant, mood stabilizer, migraine prophylaxis, voltage-sensitive sodium channel modulator

Commonly Prescribed For
(bold for FDA approved)
- **Acute mania (divalproex) and mixed episodes (divalproex, divalproex ER)**
- **Complex partial seizures that occur either in isolation or in association with other types of seizures (monotherapy and adjunctive)**
- **Simple and complex absence seizures (monotherapy and adjunctive)**
- **Multiple seizure types which include absence seizures (adjunctive)**
- **Migraine prophylaxis (divalproex, divalproex ER)**
- Maintenance treatment of bipolar disorder
- Bipolar depression
- Psychosis, schizophrenia (adjunctive)

 How The Drug Works
* Blocks voltage-sensitive sodium channels by an unknown mechanism
- Increases brain concentrations of gamma-aminobutyric acid (GABA) by an unknown mechanism

How Long Until It Works
- For acute mania, effects should occur within a few days depending on the formulation of the drug
- May take several weeks to months to optimize an effect on mood stabilization
- Should also reduce seizures and improve migraine within a few weeks

If It Works
- The goal of treatment is complete remission of symptoms (e.g., mania, seizures, migraine)

- Continue treatment until all symptoms are gone or until improvement is stable and then continue treating indefinitely as long as improvement persists
- Continue treatment indefinitely to avoid recurrence of mania, depression, seizures, and headaches

If It Doesn't Work (for bipolar disorder)
* Many patients only have a partial response where some symptoms are improved but others persist or continue to wax and wane without stabilization of mood
- Other patients may be nonresponders, sometimes called treatment-resistant or treatment-refractory
- Consider checking plasma drug level, increasing dose, switching to another agent or adding an appropriate augmenting agent
- Consider adding psychotherapy
- Consider the presence of noncompliance and counsel patient
- Switch to another mood stabilizer with fewer side effects
- Consider evaluation for another diagnosis or for a comorbid condition (e.g., medical illness, substance abuse, etc.)

 Best Augmenting Combos for Partial Response or Treatment-Resistance (for bipolar disorder)
- Lithium
- Atypical antipsychotics (especially risperidone, olanzapine, quetiapine, ziprasidone, and aripiprazole)
* Lamotrigine (with caution and at half the dose in the presence of valproate because valproate can double lamotrigine levels)
* Antidepressants (with caution because antidepressants can destabilize mood in some patients, including induction of rapid cycling or suicidal ideation; in particular consider bupropion; also SSRIs, SNRIs, others; generally avoid TCAs, MAOIs)

Tests
* Before starting treatment, platelet counts and liver function tests
- Consider coagulation tests prior to planned surgery or if there is a history of bleeding

• During the first few months of treatment, regular liver function tests and platelet counts; this can be shifted to once or twice a year for the remainder of treatment

• Plasma drug levels can assist monitoring of efficacy, side effects, and compliance

✳ Since valproate is frequently associated with weight gain, before starting treatment, weigh all patients and determine if the patient is already overweight (BMI 25.0–29.9) or obese (BMI ≥30)

• Before giving a drug that can cause weight gain to an overweight or obese patient, consider determining whether the patient already has pre-diabetes (fasting plasma glucose 100–125 mg/dl), diabetes (fasting plasma glucose >126 mg/dl), or dyslipidemia (increased total cholesterol, LDL cholesterol and triglycerides; decreased HDL cholesterol), and treat or refer such patients for treatment, including nutrition and weight management, physical activity counseling, smoking cessation, and medical management

✳ Monitor weight and BMI during treatment

✳ While giving a drug to a patient who has gained >5% of initial weight, consider evaluating for the presence of pre-diabetes, diabetes, or dyslipidemia, or consider switching to a different agent

SIDE EFFECTS

How Drug Causes Side Effects

• CNS side effects theoretically due to excessive actions at voltage-sensitive sodium channels

Notable Side Effects

✳ Sedation, tremor, dizziness, ataxia, asthenia, headache

✳ Abdominal pain, nausea, vomiting, diarrhea, reduced appetite, constipation, dyspepsia, weight gain

✳ Alopecia (unusual)

• Polycystic ovaries (controversial)

• Hyperandrogenism, hyperinsulinemia, lipid dysregulation (controversial)

• Decreased bone mineral density (controversial)

Life Threatening or Dangerous Side Effects

• Rare hepatotoxicity with liver failure sometimes severe and fatal, particularly in children under 2

• Rare pancreatitis, sometimes fatal

Weight Gain

unusual not unusual common problematic

• Many experience and/or can be significant in amount

• Can become a health problem in some

Sedation

unusual not unusual common problematic

• Frequent and can be significant in amount

• Some patients may not tolerate it

• Can wear off over time

• Can reemerge as dose increases and then wear off again over time

What To Do About Side Effects

• Wait

• Wait

• Wait

• Take at night to reduce daytime sedation, especially with divalproex ER

• Lower the dose

• Switch to another agent

Best Augmenting Agents for Side Effects

✳ Propranolol 20–30 mg 2–3 times/day may reduce tremor

✳ Multivitamins fortified with zinc and selenium may help reduce alopecia

• Many side effects cannot be improved with an augmenting agent

DOSING AND USE

Usual Dosage Range

• Mania: 1200–1500 mg/day

• Migraine: 500–1000 mg/day

• Epilepsy: 10–60 mg/kg/day

Dosage Forms

• Tablet [delayed release, as divalproex sodium (Depakote)] 125 mg, 250 mg, 500 mg

- Tablet [extended release, as divalproex sodium (Depakote ER)] 250 mg, 500 mg
- Capsule [sprinkle, as divalproex sodium (Depakote Sprinkle)] 125 mg
- Capsule [as valproic acid (Depakene)] 250 mg
- Injection [as sodium valproate (Depacon)] 100 mg/mL (5 mL)
- Syrup [as sodium valproate (Depakene)] 250 mg/5mL (5 mL, 50 mL, 480 mL)

How to Dose

- Usual starting dose for mania or epilepsy is 15 mg/kg in 2 divided doses (once daily for extended release valproate)
- Acute mania (adults): initial 1000 mg/day; increase dose rapidly; maximum dose generally 60 mg/kg/day
- For less acute mania, may begin at 250–500 mg the first day, and then titrate upward as tolerated
- Migraine (adults): initial 500 mg/day, maximum recommended dose 1000 mg/day
- Epilepsy (adults): initial 10–15 mg/kg/day; increase by 5–10 mg/kg/week; maximum dose generally 60 mg/kg/day

 Dosing Tips

* Oral loading with 20–30 mg/kg/day may reduce onset of action to 5 days or less and may be especially useful for treatment of acute mania in inpatient settings
- Given the half-life of immediate release valproate (e.g., Depakene, Depakote), twice daily dosing is probably ideal
- Extended release valproate (e.g., Depakote ER) can be given once daily
- However, extended release valproate is only about 80% as bioavailable as immediate release valproate, producing plasma drug levels 10–20% lower than with immediate release valproate
* Thus, extended release valproate is dosed approximately 8–20% higher when converting patients to the ER formulation
- Depakote (divalproex sodium) is an enteric-coated stable compound containing both valproic acid and sodium valproate
* Divalproex immediate release formulation reduces gastrointestinal side effects compared to generic valproate

* Divalproex ER improves gastrointestinal side effects and alopecia compared to immediate release divalproex or generic valproate
- The amide of valproic acid is available in Europe [valpromide (Depamide)]
- Trough plasma drug levels >45 µg/ml may be required for either antimanic effects or anticonvulsant actions
- Trough plasma drug levels up to 100 µg/ml are generally well tolerated
- Trough plasma drug levels up to 125 µg/ml may be required in some acutely manic patients
- Dosages to achieve therapeutic plasma levels vary widely, often between 750–3000 mg/day

Overdose

- Fatalities have been reported; coma, restlessness, hallucinations, sedation, heart block

Long-Term Use

- Requires regular liver function tests and platelet counts

Habit Forming

- No

How to Stop

- Taper; may need to adjust dosage of concurrent medications as valproate is being discontinued
- Patients may seize upon withdrawal, especially if withdrawal is abrupt
* Rapid discontinuation increases the risk of relapse in bipolar disorder
- Discontinuation symptoms uncommon

Pharmacokinetics

- Mean terminal half-life 9–16 hours
- Metabolized primarily by the liver, approximately 25% dependent upon CYP450 system

 Drug Interactions

* Lamotrigine dose should be reduced by perhaps 50% if used with valproate, as valproate inhibits metabolism of lamotrigine and raises lamotrigine plasma levels, theoretically increasing the risk of rash

- Plasma levels of valproate may be <u>lowered</u> by carbamazepine, phenytoin, ethosuximide, phenobarbital, rifampin
- Aspirin may inhibit metabolism of valproate and <u>increase</u> valproate plasma levels
- Plasma levels of valproate may also be <u>increased</u> by felbamate, chlorpromazine, fluoxetine, fluvoxamine, topiramate, cimetidine, erythromycin, and ibuprofen
- Valproate inhibits metabolism of ethosuximide, phenobarbital, and phenytoin, and can thus <u>increase</u> their plasma levels
- No likely pharmacokinetic interactions of valproate with lithium or atypical antipsychotics
- Use of valproate with clonazepam may cause absence status

 Other Warnings/ Precautions

* Be alert to the following symptoms of hepatotoxicity that require immediate attention: malaise, weakness, lethargy, facial edema, anorexia, vomiting, yellowing of the skin and eyes
* Be alert to the following symptoms of pancreatitis that require immediate attention: abdominal pain, nausea, vomiting, anorexia
* Teratogenic effects in developing fetuses such as neural tube defects may occur with valproate use
* Somnolence may be more common in the elderly and may be associated with dehydration, reduced nutritional intake, and weight loss, requiring slower dosage increases, lower doses, and monitoring of fluid and nutritional intake
- Use in patients with thrombocytopenia is not recommended; patients should report easy bruising or bleeding
- Evaluate for urea cycle disorders, as hyperammonemic encephalopathy, sometimes fatal, has been associated with valproate administration in these uncommon disorders; urea cycle disorders, such as ormithine transcarbamylase deficiency, are associated with unexplained encephalopathy, mental retardation, elevated plasma ammonia, cyclical vomiting, and lethargy

Do Not Use
- If patient has pancreatitis
- If patient has serious liver disease
- If patient has urea cycle disorder
- If there is a proven allergy to valproic acid, valproate, or divalproex

SPECIAL POPULATIONS

Renal Impairment
- No dose adjustment necessary

Hepatic Impairment
- Contraindicated

Cardiac Impairment
- No dose adjustment necessary

Elderly
- Reduce starting dose and titrate slowly; dosing is generally lower than in healthy adults
* Sedation in the elderly may be more common and associated with dehydration, reduced nutritional intake, and weight loss
- Monitor fluid and nutritional intake

 Children and Adolescents

* Not generally recommended for use under age 10 for bipolar disorder except by experts and when other options have been considered
- Children under age 2 have significantly increased risk of hepatotoxicity, as they have a markedly decreased ability to eliminate valproate compared to older children and adults
- Use requires close medical supervision

 Pregnancy
- Risk category D [positive evidence of risk to human fetus; potential benefits may still justify its use during pregnancy]
* Use during first trimester may raise risk of neural tube defects (e.g., spina bifida) or other congenital anomalies
- Use in women of childbearing potential requires weighing potential benefits to the mother against the risks to the fetus

* If drug is continued, monitor clotting parameters and perform tests to detect birth defects
* If drug is continued, start on folate 1 mg/day early in pregnancy to reduce risk of neural tube defects
* If drug is continued, consider vitamin K during the last 6 weeks of pregnancy to reduce risks of bleeding
* Antiepileptic Drug Pregnancy Registry: (888) 233-2334
* Taper drug if discontinuing
* Seizures, even mild seizures, may cause harm to the embryo/fetus
* For bipolar patients, valproate should generally be discontinued before anticipated pregnancies
* Recurrent bipolar illness during pregnancy can be quite disruptive
* For bipolar patients, given the risk of relapse in the postpartum period, mood stabilizer treatment such as valproate should generally be restarted immediately after delivery if patient is unmedicated during pregnancy
* Atypical antipsychotics may be preferable to lithium or anticonvulsants such as valproate if treatment of bipolar disorder is required during pregnancy
* Bipolar symptoms may recur or worsen during pregnancy and some form of treatment may be necessary

Breast Feeding

* Some drug is found in mother's breast milk
* Generally considered safe to breast feed while taking valproate
* If drug is continued while breast feeding, infant should be monitored for possible adverse effects
* If infant shows signs of irritability or sedation, drug may need to be discontinued
* Bipolar disorder may recur during the postpartum period, particularly if there is a history of prior postpartum episodes of either depression or psychosis
* Relapse rates may be lower in women who receive prophylactic treatment for postpartum episodes of bipolar disorder
* Atypical antipsychotics and anticonvulsants such as valproate may be safer than lithium during the postpartum period when breast feeding

THE ART OF PSYCHOPHARMACOLOGY

Potential Advantages

* Manic phase of bipolar disorder
* Works well in combination with lithium and/or atypical antipsychotics
* Patients for whom therapeutic drug monitoring is desirable

Potential Disadvantages

* Depressed phase of bipolar disorder
* Patients unable to tolerate sedation or weight gain
* Multiple drug interactions
* Multiple side effect risks
* Pregnant patients

Primary Target Symptoms

* Unstable mood
* Incidence of migraine
* Incidence of partial complex seizures

 Pearls (for bipolar disorder)

* Valproate is a first-line treatment option that may be best for patients with mixed states of bipolar disorder or for patients with rapid-cycling bipolar disorder
* Seems to be more effective in treating manic episodes than depressive episodes in bipolar disorder (treats from above better than it treats from below)
* May also be more effective in preventing manic relapses than in preventing depressive episodes (stabilizes from above better than it stabilizes from below)
* Only a third of bipolar patients experience adequate relief with a monotherapy, so most patients need multiple medications for best control
* Useful in combination with atypical antipsychotics and/or lithium for acute mania
* May also be useful for bipolar disorder in combination with lamotrigine, but must reduce lamotrigine dose by half when combined with valproate
* Usefulness for bipolar disorder in combination with anticonvulsants other than lamotrigine is not well demonstrated; such combinations can be expensive and are possibly ineffective or even irrational
* May be useful as an adjunct to atypical antipsychotics for rapid onset of action in schizophrenia

✳ Used to treat aggression, agitation, and impulsivity not only in bipolar disorder and schizophrenia but also in many other disorders, including dementia, personality disorders, and brain injury

• Patients with acute mania tend to tolerate side effects better than patients with hypomania or depression

• Multivitamins fortified with zinc and selenium may help reduce alopecia

• Association of valproate with polycystic ovaries is controversial and may be related to weight gain, obesity, or epilepsy

• Nevertheless, may wish to be cautious in administering valproate to women of child bearing potential, especially adolescent female bipolar patients, and carefully monitor weight, endocrine status, and ovarian size and function

✳ In women of child bearing potential who are or are likely to become sexually active, should inform about risk of harm to the fetus and monitor contraceptive status

• Association of valproate with decreased bone mass is controversial and may be related to activity levels, exposure to sunlight, and epilepsy, and might be prevented by supplemental vitamin D 2000 Iu/day and calcium 600–1000 mg/day

 Suggested Reading

Bowden CL. Valproate. Bipolar Disorders 2003;5:189–202.

Emilien G, Maloteaux JM, Seghers A, Charles G. Lithium compared to valproic acid and carbamazepine in the treatment of mania: a statistical meta-analysis. Eur Neuropsychopharmacol. 1996;6:245–52.

Landy SH, McGinnis J. Divalproex sodium—review of prophylactic migraine efficacy, safety and dosage, with recommendations. Tenn Med. 1999;92:135–6.

Macritchie KA, Geddes JR, Scott J, Haslam DR, Goodwin GM. Valproic acid, valproate and divalproex in the maintenance treatment of bipolar disorder. Cochrane Database Syst Rev. 2001;(3):CD003196.

Strakowski SM, DelBello MP, Adler CM. Comparative efficacy and tolerability of drug treatments for bipolar disorder. CNS Drugs. 2001;15:701–18.

ZIPRASIDONE

THERAPEUTICS

Brands • Geodon
see index for additional brand names

Generic? Not in U.S. or Europe

Class

• Atypical antipsychotic (serotonin-dopamine antagonist; second generation antipsychotic; also a mood stabilizer)

Commonly Prescribed For
(bold for FDA approved)

• **Schizophrenia**
• **Delaying relapse in schizophrenia**
• **Acute agitation in schizophrenia (intramuscular)**
• **Acute mania/mixed mania**
• Other psychotic disorders
• Bipolar maintenance
• Bipolar depression
• Behavioral disturbances in dementias
• Behavioral disturbances in children and adolescents
• Disorders associated with problems with impulse control

How The Drug Works

• Blocks dopamine 2 receptors, reducing positive symptoms of psychosis and stabilizing affective symptoms
• Blocks serotonin 2A receptors, causing enhancement of dopamine release in certain brain regions and thus reducing motor side effects and possibly improving cognitive and affective symptoms
• Interactions at a myriad of other neurotransmitter receptors may contribute to ziprasidone's efficacy
✳ Specifically, interactions at 5HT2C and 5HT1A receptors may contribute to efficacy for cognitive and affective symptoms in some patients
✳ Specifically, interactions at 5HT1D receptors and at serotonin, norepinephrine, and dopamine transporters (especially at high doses) may contribute to efficacy for affective symptoms in some patients

How Long Until It Works

• Psychotic and manic symptoms can improve within 1 week, but it may take several weeks for full effect on behavior as well as on cognition and affective stabilization
• Classically recommended to wait at least 4–6 weeks to determine efficacy of drug, but in practice some patients require up to 16–20 weeks to show a good response, especially on cognitive symptoms
• IM formulation can reduce agitation in 15 minutes

If It Works

• Most often reduces positive symptoms in schizophrenia but does not eliminate them
• Can improve negative symptoms, as well as aggressive, cognitive, and affective symptoms in schizophrenia
• Most schizophrenic patients do not have a total remission of symptoms but rather a reduction of symptoms by about a third
• Perhaps 5–15% of schizophrenic patients can experience an overall improvement of greater than 50–60%, especially when receiving stable treatment for more than a year
• Such patients are considered super-responders or "awakeners" since they may be well enough to be employed, live independently, and sustain long-term relationships
• Many bipolar patients may experience a reduction of symptoms by half or more
• Continue treatment until reaching a plateau of improvement
• After reaching a satisfactory plateau, continue treatment for at least a year after first episode of psychosis
• For second and subsequent episodes of psychosis, treatment may need to be indefinite
• Even for first episodes of psychosis, it may be preferable to continue treatment indefinitely to avoid subsequent episodes
• Treatment may not only reduce mania but also prevent recurrences of mania in bipolar disorder

If It Doesn't Work

• Try one of the other atypical antipsychotics (risperidone, olanzapine, quetiapine, aripiprazole, amisulpride)
• If 2 or more antipsychotic monotherapies do not work, consider clozapine

- If no first-line atypical antipsychotic is effective, consider higher doses or augmentation with valproate or lamotrigine
- Some patients may require treatment with a conventional antipsychotic
- Consider noncompliance and switch to another antipsychotic with fewer side effects or to an antipsychotic that can be given by depot injection
- Consider initiating rehabilitation and psychotherapy
- Consider presence of concomitant drug abuse

 ### Best Augmenting Combos for Partial Response or Treatment-Resistance

- Valproic acid (valproate, divalproex, divalproex ER)
- Other mood stabilizing anticonvulsants (carbamazepine, oxcarbazepine, lamotrigine)
- Lithium
- Benzodiazepines

Tests

Before starting an atypical antipsychotic

* Weigh all patients and track BMI during treatment
- Get baseline personal and family history of diabetes, obesity, dyslipidemia, hypertension, and cardiovascular disease
* Get waist circumference (at umbilicus), blood pressure, fasting plasma glucose, and fasting lipid profile
- Determine if the patient is
  - overweight (BMI 25.0–29.9)
  - obese (BMI ≥30)
  - has pre-diabetes (fasting plasma glucose 100–125 mg/dl)
  - has diabetes (fasting plasma glucose >126 mg/dl)
  - has hypertension (BP >140/90 mm Hg)
  - has dyslipidemia (increased total cholesterol, LDL cholesterol, and triglycerides; decreased HDL cholesterol)
- Treat or refer such patients for treatment, including nutrition and weight management, physical activity counseling, smoking cessation, and medical management

Monitoring after starting an atypical antipsychotic

* BMI monthly for 3 months, then quarterly

* Blood pressure, fasting plasma glucose, fasting lipids within 3 months and then annually, but earlier and more frequently for patients with diabetes or who have gained >5% of initial weight
- Treat or refer for treatment and consider switching to another atypical antipsychotic for patients who become overweight, obese, pre-diabetic, diabetic, hypertensive, or dyslipidemic while receiving an atypical antipsychotic
* Even in patients without known diabetes, be vigilant for the rare but life threatening onset of diabetic ketoacidosis, which always requires immediate treatment, by monitoring for the rapid onset of polyuria, polydipsia, weight loss, nausea, vomiting, dehydration, rapid respiration, weakness and clouding of sensorium, even coma
- Routine EKGs for screening or monitoring of dubious clinical value
- EKGs may be useful for selected patients (e.g., those with personal or family history of QTc prolongation; cardiac arrhythmia; recent myocardial infarction; uncompensated heart failure; or those taking agents that prolong QTc interval such as pimozide, thioridazine, selected antiarrhythmics, moxifloxacin, sparfloxacin, etc.)
- Patients at risk for electrolyte disturbances (e.g., patients on diuretic therapy) should have baseline and periodic serum potassium and magnesium measurements

SIDE EFFECTS

How Drug Causes Side Effects

- By blocking alpha 1 adrenergic receptors, it can cause dizziness, sedation, and hypotension, especially at high doses
- By blocking dopamine 2 receptors in the striatum, it can cause motor side effects (unusual)
* Mechanism of any possible weight gain is unknown; weight gain is not common with ziprasidone and may thus have a different mechanism from atypical antipsychotics for which weight gain is common or problematic
* Mechanism of any possible increased incidence of diabetes or dyslipidemia is unknown; early experience suggests these

complications are not clearly associated with ziprasidone and if present may therefore have a different mechanism from that of atypical antipsychotics associated with an increased incidence of diabetes and dyslipidemia

Notable Side Effects

* ❋ Some patients may experience activating side effects at very low to low doses
* Dizziness, extrapyramidal symptoms, sedation, dystonia at high doses
* Nausea, dry mouth
* Asthenia, skin rash
* Rare tardive dyskinesia (much reduced risk compared to conventional antipsychotics)
* Orthostatic hypotension

 ## Life Threatening or Dangerous Side Effects

* Rare neuroleptic malignant syndrome (much reduced risk compared to conventional antipsychotics)
* Rare seizures
* Increased risk of death and cerebrovascular events in elderly patients with dementia-related psychosis

Weight Gain

unusual   not unusual   common   problematic

* Reported in a few patients, especially those with low BMIs, but not expected
* Less frequent and less severe than for most other antipsychotics

Sedation

unusual   not unusual   common   problematic

* Some patients experience, especially at high doses
* May be less than for some antipsychotics, more than for others
* Usually transient and at higher doses
* Can be activating at low doses

What To Do About Side Effects

* Wait
* Wait
* Wait
* Usually dosed twice daily, so take more of the total daily dose at bedtime to help reduce daytime sedation

* Anticholinergics may reduce motor side effects when present
* Weight loss, exercise programs, and medical management for high BMIs, diabetes, dyslipidemia
* ❋ For activating side effects at low doses, raise the dose
* ❋ For sedating side effects at high doses, lower the dose
* Switch to another atypical antipsychotic

Best Augmenting Agents for Side Effects

* Benztropine or trihexyphenidyl for motor side effects
* Many side effects cannot be improved with an augmenting agent

DOSING AND USE

Usual Dosage Range

* Schizophrenia: 40–200 mg/day (in divided doses) orally
* Bipolar disorder: 80–160 mg/day (in divided doses) orally
* 10–20 mg intramuscularly

Dosage Forms

* Capsules 20 mg, 40 mg, 60 mg, 80 mg
* Injection 20 mg/mL

How to Dose

* Schizophrenia (according to manufacturer): initial oral dose 20 mg twice a day; however, 40 mg twice a day or 60 mg twice a day may be better tolerated in many patients (less activation); maximum approved dose 100 mg twice a day
* Biplar disorder (according to manufacturer): initial oral dose 40 mg twice a day; on day 2 increase to 60 or 80 mg twice a day
* For intramuscular formulation, recommended dose is 10–20 mg given as required; doses of 10 mg may be administered every 2 hours; doses of 20 mg may be administered every 4 hours; maximum daily dose 40 mg intramuscularly; should not be administered for more than 3 consecutive days

Dosing Tips

✷ **More may be much more:** clinical practice suggests ziprasidone often under-dosed, then switched prior to adequate trials, perhaps due to unjustified fears of QTc prolongation

✷ Dosing many patients at 20–40 mg twice a day is too low and in fact activating, perhaps due to potent 5HT2C antagonist properties

✷ Paradoxically, such activation is often reduced by increasing the dose to 60–80 mg twice a day, perhaps due to increasing amounts of dopamine 2 receptor antagonism

✷ Best efficacy in schizophrenia and bipolar disorder is at doses >120 mg/day, but only a minority of patients are adequately dosed in clinical practice

• Doses up to 80 mg twice a day may have a lower cost than some other atypical antipsychotics

• Intramuscular formulation costs about the same as haloperidol injections

✷ Recommended to be taken with food because food can double bioavailability by increasing absorption and thus increasing plasma drug levels

• Some patients respond better to doses >160 mg/day and up to 320 mg/day in 2 divided doses (i.e., 80–160 mg twice a day)

• Many patients do well with a single daily oral dose, usually at bedtime

• Although studies suggest patients switching to ziprasidone from another antipsychotic can do well with rapid cross-titration, clinical experience suggests many patients do best by building up a full dose of ziprasidone (>120 mg/day) added to the maintenance dose of the first antipsychotic for up to 3 weeks prior to slow down-titration of the first antipsychotic

• QTc prolongation at 320 mg/day not significantly greater than at 160 mg/day

• Rather than raise the dose above these levels in acutely agitated patients requiring acute antipsychotic actions, consider augmentation with a benzodiazepine or conventional antipsychotic, either orally or intramuscularly

• Rather than raise the dose above these levels in partial responders, consider augmentation with a mood stabilizing anticonvulsant, such as valproate or lamotrigine

• Children and elderly should generally be dosed at the lower end of the dosage spectrum

• Ziprasidone intramuscular can be given short-term, both to initiate dosing with oral ziprasidone or another oral antipsychotic and to treat breakthrough agitation in patients maintained on oral antipsychotics

• QTc prolongation of intramuscular ziprasidone is the same or less than with intramuscular haloperidol

Overdose

• Rarely lethal in monotherapy overdose; sedation, slurred speech, transitory hypertension

Long-Term Use

• Approved to delay relapse in long-term treatment of schizophrenia

• Often used for long-term maintenance in bipolar disorder and various behavioral disorders

Habit Forming

• No

How to Stop

• Slow down-titration of oral formulation (over 6 to 8 weeks), especially when simultaneously beginning a new antipsychotic while switching (i.e. cross-titration)

• Rapid oral discontinuation may lead to rebound psychosis and worsening of symptoms

Pharmacokinetics

• Mean half-life 6.6 hours
• Protein binding >99%
• Metabolized by CYP450 3A4

 Drug Interactions

• Neither CYP450 3A4 nor CYP450 2D6 inhibitors significantly affect ziprasidone plasma levels

• Little potential to affect metabolism of drugs cleared by CYP450 enzymes

• May enhance the effects of antihypertensive drugs

• May antagonize levodopa, dopamine agonists
• May enhance QTc prolongation of other drugs capable of prolonging QTc interval

 Other Warnings/ Precautions

• Ziprasidone prolongs QTc interval more than some other antipsychotics
• Use with caution in patients with conditions that predispose to hypotension (dehydration, overheating)
• Priapism has been reported
• Dysphagia has been associated with antipsychotic use, and ziprasidone should be used cautiously in patients at risk for aspiration pneumonia

Do Not Use

• If patient is taking agents capable of significantly prolonging QTc interval (e.g., pimozide, thioridazine, selected antiarrhythmics, moxifloxacin, sparfloxacin)
• If there is a history of QTc prolongation or cardiac arrhythmia, recent acute myocardial infarction, uncompensated heart failure
• If there is a proven allergy to ziprasidone

SPECIAL POPULATIONS

Renal Impairment

• No dose adjustment necessary
• Not removed by hemodialysis
• Intramuscular formulation should be used with caution

Hepatic Impairment

• No dose adjustment necessary

Cardiac Impairment

• Ziprasidone is contraindicated in patients with a known history of QTc prolongation, recent acute myocardial infarction, and uncompensated heart failure
• Should be used with caution in other cases of cardiac impairment because of risk of orthostatic hypotension

Elderly

• Some patients may tolerate lower doses better

• Although atypical antipsychotics are commonly used for behavioral disturbances in dementia, no agent has been approved for treatment of elderly patients with dementia-related psychosis
• Elderly patients with dementia-related psychosis treated with atypical antipsychotics are at an increased risk of death compared to placebo, and also have an increased risk of cerebrovascular events

 Children and Adolescents

• Not officially recommended for patients under age 18
• Clinical experience and early data suggest ziprasidone may be safe and effective for behavioral disturbances in children and adolescents
• Children and adolescents using ziprasidone may need to be monitored more often than adults and may tolerate lower doses better

 Pregnancy

• Risk Category C [some animal studies show adverse effects, no controlled studies in humans]
• Psychotic symptoms may worsen during pregnancy and some form of treatment may be necessary
• Ziprasidone may be preferable to anticonvulsant mood stabilizers if treatment is required during pregnancy

Breast Feeding

• Unknown if ziprasidone is secreted in human breast milk, but all psychotropics assumed to be secreted in breast milk
✳ Recommended either to discontinue drug or bottle feed
• Infants of women who choose to breast feed while on ziprasidone should be monitored for possible adverse effects

THE ART OF PSYCHOPHARMACOLOGY

Potential Advantages

• Some cases of psychosis and bipolar disorder refractory to treatment with other antipsychotics

✳ Patients concerned about gaining weight and patients who are already obese or overweight
✳ Patients with diabetes
✳ Patients with dyslipidemia (especially elevated triglycerides)
• Patients requiring rapid relief of symptoms (intramuscular injection)
• Patients switching from intramuscular ziprasidone to an oral preparation

Potential Disadvantages

• Patients noncompliant with twice daily dosing
✳ Patients noncompliant with dosing with food

Primary Target Symptoms

• Positive symptoms of psychosis
• Negative symptoms of psychosis
• Cognitive symptoms
• Unstable mood (both depression and mania)
• Aggressive symptoms

 Pearls

• Recent landmark head to head study in schizophrenia suggests lower metabolic side effects and comparable efficacy compared to some other atypical and conventional antipsychotics
✳ When given to patients with obesity and dyslipidemia associated with prior treatment with another atypical antipsychotic, many experience weight loss and decrease in fasting triglycerides
✳ QTc prolongation fears are often exaggerated and not justified since QTc prolongation with ziprasidone is not dose-related and few drugs have any potential to increase ziprasidone's plasma levels
✳ Efficacy may be underestimated since ziprasidone is mostly under-dosed (<120 mg/day) in clinical practice
✳ Well-accepted in clinical practice when wanting to avoid weight gain because less weight gain than most other atypical antipsychotics
✳ May not have diabetes or dyslipidemia risk, but monitoring is still indicated
• Less sedation than some antipsychotics, more than others (at moderate to high doses)
✳ More activating than some other antipsychotics at low doses
• One of the least expensive atypical antipsychotics within recommended therapeutic dosing range
• Anecdotal reports of utility in treatment-resistant cases, especially when adequately dosed
✳ One of only 2 atypical antipsychotics with a short-acting intramuscular dosage formulation

 Suggested Reading

Bantick RA, Deakin JF, Grasby PM. The 5-HT1A receptor in schizophrenia: a promising target for novel atypical neuroleptics? J Psychopharmacol 2001;15:37–46.

Gunasekara NS, Spencer CM, Keating GM. Spotlight on ziprasidone in schizophrenia and schizoaffective disorder. CNS Drugs 2002;16:645–52.

Keck PE Jr, McElroy SL, Arnold LM. Ziprasidone: a new atypical antipsychotic. Expert Opin Pharmacother 2001;2:1033–42.

Lieberman JA, Stroup TS, McEvoy JP, Swartz MS, Rosenheck RA, Perkins DO et al. Effectiveness of antipsychotic drugs in patients with chronic schizophrenia. N Engl J Med 2005;353(12):1209–23.

Taylor D. Ziprasidone in the management of schizophrenia : the QT interval issue in context. CNS Drugs 2003;17:423–30.

Yatham LN. Efficacy of atypical antipsychotics in mood disorders. J Clin Psychopharmacol 2003;23(3 Suppl 1):S9–14.

ZONISAMIDE

THERAPEUTICS

Brands
- Zonegran
- Excegran

see index for additional brand names

Generic? Not in U.S.

 Class
- Anticonvulsant, voltage-sensitive sodium channel modulator; T-type calcium channel modulator; structurally a sulfonamide

Commonly Prescribed For
(bold for FDA approved)
- **Adjunct therapy for partial seizures in adults with epilepsy**
- Bipolar disorder
- Chronic neuropathic pain
- Migraine
- Parkinson's disease
- Psychotropic drug-induced weight gain
- Binge-eating disorder

 How The Drug Works
- Unknown
- Modulates voltage-sensitive sodium channels by an unknown mechanism
- Also modulates T-type calcium channels
- Facilitates dopamine and serotonin release
- Inhibits carbonic anhydrase

How Long Until It Works
- Should reduce seizures by 2 weeks
- Onset of action as well as convincing therapeutic efficacy have not been demonstrated for uses other than adjunctive treatment of partial seizures

If It Works
- The goal of treatment is complete remission of symptoms (e.g., seizures, pain, mania, migraine)
- Would currently only be expected to work in a subset of patients for conditions other than epilepsy as an adjunctive treatment to agents with better demonstration of efficacy

If It Doesn't Work (for conditions other than epilepsy)
- May only be effective in patients who fail to respond to agents with proven efficacy, or it may not work at all
- Consider increasing dose or switching to another agent with better demonstrated efficacy

 Best Augmenting Combos for Partial Response or Treatment-Resistance
- Zonisamide is itself a second-line augmenting agent to numerous other agents in treating conditions other than epilepsy, such as bipolar disorder, chronic neuropathic pain, and migraine

Tests
- Consider baseline and periodic monitoring of renal function

SIDE EFFECTS

How Drug Causes Side Effects
- CNS side effects theoretically due to excessive actions at voltage-sensitive ion channels
- Weak inhibition of carbonic anhydrase may lead to kidney stones
- Serious rash theoretically an allergic reaction

Notable Side Effects
* Sedation, depression, difficulty concentrating, agitation, irritability, psychomotor slowing, dizziness, ataxia
- Headache
- Nausea, anorexia, abdominal pain, vomiting
- Kidney stones
- Elevated serum creatinine and blood urea nitrogen

 Life Threatening or Dangerous Side Effects
- Rare serious rash (Stevens Johnson syndrome, toxic epidermal necrolysis) (sulfonamide)
- Rare oligohidrosis and hyperthermia (pediatric patients)
- Rare blood dyscrasias (aplastic anemia; agranulocytosis)
- Sudden hepatic necrosis

• Sudden unexplained deaths have occurred (unknown if related to zonisamide use)

Weight Gain

unusual   not unusual   common   problematic

• Reported but not expected
✱ Patients may experience weight loss

Sedation

unusual   not unusual   common   problematic

• Many experience and/or can be significant in amount
• Dose-related
• Can wear off with time but may not wear off at high doses

What To Do About Side Effects

• Wait
• Wait
• Wait
• Take more of the dose at night to reduce daytime sedation
• Lower the dose
• Switch to another agent

Best Augmenting Agents for Side Effects

• Many side effects cannot be improved with an augmenting agent

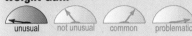

DOSING AND USE

Usual Dosage Range

• 100–600 mg/day in 1–2 doses

Dosage Forms

• Capsule 25 mg, 50 mg, 100 mg

How to Dose

• Initial 100 mg/day; after 2 weeks can increase to 200 mg/day; dose can be increased by 100 mg/day every 2 weeks if necessary and tolerated; maximum dose generally 600 mg/day; maintain stable dose for at least 2 weeks before increasing dose

 Dosing Tips

✱ Most clinical experience is at doses up to 400 mg/day

• No evidence from controlled trials of increasing response over 400 mg/day
• However, some patients may tolerate and respond to doses up to 600 mg/day
• Little experience with doses greater than 600 mg/day
• Side effects may increase notably at doses greater than 300 mg/day
• For intolerable sedation, can give most of the dose at night and less during the day

Overdose

• Can cause bradycardia, hypotension, respiratory depression

Long-Term Use

• Safe
• Consider periodic monitoring of blood urea nitrogen and creatinine

Habit Forming

• No

How to Stop

• Taper
• Epilepsy patients may seize upon withdrawal, especially if withdrawal is abrupt
• Rapid discontinuation may increase the risk of relapse in bipolar patients
• Discontinuation symptoms uncommon

Pharmacokinetics

• Plasma elimination half-life approximately 63 hours
• Metabolized in part by CYP450 3A4
• Partially eliminated renally

 Drug Interactions

• Agents that inhibit CYP450 3A4 (such as nefazodone, fluvoxamine, and fluoxetine) may decrease the clearance of zonisamide, and increase plasma zonisamide levels, possibly requiring lower doses of zonisamide
• Agents that induce CYP450 3A4 (such as carbamazepine) may increase the clearance of zonisamide and decrease plasma zonisamide levels, possibly requiring higher doses of zonisamide
• Enzyme-inducing antiepileptic drugs (carbamazepine, phenytoin, phenobarbital, and primidone) may decrease plasma levels of zonisamide

• Theoretically, zonisamide may interact with carbonic anhydrase inhibitors to increase the risk of kidney stones

 ### Other Warnings/ Precautions

• Depressive effects may be increased by other CNS depressants (alcohol, MAOIs, other anticonvulsants, etc.)
• Use with caution when combining with other drugs that predispose patients to heat-related disorders, including carbonic anhydrase inhibitors and anticholinergics
✳ Life-threatening rashes have developed in association with zonisamide use; zonisamide should generally be discontinued at the first sign of serious rash
• Patient should be instructed to report any symptoms of hypersensitivity immediately (fever; flu-like symptoms; rash; blisters on skin or in eyes, mouth, ears, nose, or genital areas; swelling of eyelids, conjunctivitis, lymphadenopathy)
• Patients should be monitored for signs of unusual bleeding or bruising, mouth sores, infections, fever, and sore throat, as there may be an increased risk of aplastic anemia and agranulocytosis with zonisamide

Do Not Use

• If there is a proven allergy to zonisamide or sulfonamides

SPECIAL POPULATIONS

Renal Impairment

• Zonisamide is primarily renally excreted
• Use with caution
• May require slower titration

Hepatic Impairment

• Use with caution
• May require slower titration

Cardiac Impairment

• No specific recommendations

Elderly

• Some patients may tolerate lower doses better
• Elderly patients may be more susceptible to adverse effects

 ### Children and Adolescents

• Cases of oligohidrosis and hyperthermia have been reported
• Not approved for use in children under age 16
• Use in children for the expert only, with close monitoring, after other options have failed

Pregnancy

• Risk category C [some animal studies show adverse effects, no controlled studies in humans]
• Use in women of childbearing potential requires weighing potential benefits to the mother against the risks to the fetus
• Antiepileptic Drug Pregnancy Registry: (888) 233-2334
• Taper drug if discontinuing
• Seizures, even mild seizures, may cause harm to the embryo/fetus
• Lack of convincing efficacy for treatment of conditions other than epilepsy suggests risk/benefit ratio is in favor of discontinuing zonisamide during pregnancy for these indications

Breast Feeding

• Unknown if zonisamide is secreted in human breast milk, but all psychotropics assumed to be secreted in breast milk
✳ Recommended either to discontinue drug or bottle feed
• If drug is continued while breast feeding, infant should be monitored for possible adverse effects
• If child becomes irritable or sedated, breast feeding or drug may need to be discontinued

THE ART OF PSYCHOPHARMACOLOGY

Potential Advantages

• Treatment-resistant conditions
• Patients who wish to avoid weight gain

Potential Disadvantages

• Poor documentation of efficacy for off-label uses

- Patients noncompliant with twice daily dosing

Primary Target Symptoms

- Seizures
- Numerous other symptoms for off-label uses
- Patients with a history of kidney stones

 Pearls

- Well studied in epilepsy
- ✳ Much off-label use is based upon theoretical considerations rather than clinical experience or compelling efficacy studies
- Early studies suggest efficacy in binge-eating disorder

- Early studies suggest possible efficacy in migraine
- Early studies suggest possible utility in Parkinson's disease
- Early studies suggest possible utility in neuropathic pain
- Early studies suggest some therapeutic potential for mood stabilizing
- Chronic intake of caffeine may lower brain zonisamide concentrations and attenuate its anticonvulsant effects (based on animal studies)
- ✳ Due to reported weight loss in some patients in trials with epilepsy, some patients with psychotropic-induced weight gain are treated with zonisamide
- Utility for this indication is not clear nor has it been systematically studied

 Suggested Reading

Chadwick DW, Marson AG. Zonisamide add-on for drug-resistant partial epilepsy. Cochrane Database Syst Rev. 2002;(2):CD001416.

Glauser TA, Pellock JM. Zonisamide in pediatric epilepsy: review of the Japanese experience. J Child Neurol. 2002;17:87–96.

Jain KK. An assessment of zonisamide as an anti-epileptic drug. Expert Opin Pharmacother. 2000;1:1245–60.

Leppik IE. Three new drugs for epilepsy: levetiracetam, oxcarbazepine, and zonisamide. J Child Neurol. 2002;17 Suppl 1:S53–7.

Brands • Lodopin
• Zoleptil
see index for additional brand names

Generic? No

Class

• Atypical antipsychotic (serotonin-dopamine antagonist)

Commonly Prescribed For
(bold for FDA approved)
• Schizophrenia
• Other psychotic disorders
• Mania

How The Drug Works

• Blocks dopamine 2 receptors, reducing positive symptoms of psychosis
• Blocks serotonin 2A receptors, causing enhancement of dopamine release in certain brain regions and thus reducing motor side effects and possibly improving cognitive and affective symptoms
• Interactions at a myriad of other neurotransmitter receptors may contribute to zotepine's efficacy
* Specifically inhibits norepinephrine uptake

How Long Until It Works

• Psychotic and manic symptoms can improve within 1 week, but it may take several weeks for full effect on behavior as well as on cognition and affective stabilization
• Classically recommended to wait at least 4–6 weeks to determine efficacy of drug, but in practice some patients require up to 16–20 weeks to show a good response, especially on cognitive symptoms

If It Works

• Most often reduces positive symptoms in schizophrenia but does not eliminate them
• Can improve negative symptoms, as well as aggressive, cognitive, and affective symptoms in schizophrenia
• Most schizophrenic patients do not have a total remission of symptoms but rather a reduction of symptoms by about a third

• Perhaps 5–15% of schizophrenic patients can experience an overall improvement of greater than 50–60%, especially when receiving stable treatment for more than a year
• Such patients are considered super-responders or "awakeners" since they may be well enough to be employed, live independently, and sustain long-term relationships
• Many bipolar patients may experience a reduction of symptoms by half or more
• Continue treatment until reaching a plateau of improvement
• After reaching a satisfactory plateau, continue treatment for at least a year after first episode of psychosis
• For second and subsequent episodes of psychosis, treatment may need to be indefinite
• Even for first episodes of psychosis, it may be preferable to continue treatment indefinitely to avoid subsequent episodes
• Treatment may not only reduce mania but also prevent recurrences of mania in bipolar disorder

If It Doesn't Work

• Consider trying one of the first-line atypical antipsychotics (risperidone, olanzapine, quetiapine, ziprasidone, aripiprazole, amisulpride)
• If 2 or more antipsychotic monotherapies do not work, consider clozapine
• If no first-line atypical antipsychotic is effective, consider higher doses or augmentation with valproate or lamotrigine
• Some patients may require treatment with a conventional antipsychotic
• Consider noncompliance and switch to another antipsychotic with fewer side effects or to an antipsychotic that can be given by depot injection
• Consider initiating rehabilitation and psychotherapy
• Consider presence of concomitant drug abuse

Best Augmenting Combos for Partial Response or Treatment-Resistance

• Augmentation of zotepine has not been systematically studied
• Valproic acid (valproate, divalproex, divalproex ER)

- Other mood stabilizing anticonvulsants (carbamazepine, oxcarbazepine, lamotrigine)
- Lithium
- Benzodiazepines

Tests

❋ Although risk of diabetes and dyslipidemia with zotepine has not been systematically studied, monitoring as for all other atypical antipsychotics is suggested

Before starting an atypical antipsychotic

❋ Weigh all patients and track BMI during treatment
- Get baseline personal and family history of diabetes, obesity, dyslipidemia, hypertension, and cardiovascular disease
❋ Get waist circumference (at umbilicus), blood pressure, fasting plasma glucose, and fasting lipid profile
- Determine if the patient is
  - overweight (BMI 25.0–29.9)
  - obese (BMI ≥30)
  - has pre-diabetes (fasting plasma glucose 100–125 mg/dl)
  - has diabetes (fasting plasma glucose >126 mg/dl)
  - has hypertension (BP >140/90 mm Hg)
  - has dyslipidemia (increased total cholesterol, LDL cholesterol, and triglycerides; decreased HDL cholesterol)
- Treat or refer such patients for treatment, including nutrition and weight management, physical activity counseling, smoking cessation, and medical management

Monitoring after starting an atypical antipsychotic

❋ BMI monthly for 3 months, then quarterly
❋ Blood pressure, fasting plasma glucose, fasting lipids within 3 months and then annually, but earlier and more frequently for patients with diabetes or who have gained >5% of initial weight
- Treat or refer for treatment and consider switching to another atypical antipsychotic for patients who become overweight, obese, pre-diabetic, diabetic, hypertensive, or dyslipidemic while receiving an atypical antipsychotic
❋ Even in patients without known diabetes, be vigilant for the rare but life threatening onset of diabetic ketoacidosis, which always requires immediate treatment, by monitoring for the rapid onset of polyuria, polydipsia, weight loss, nausea, vomiting, dehydration, rapid respiration, weakness and clouding of sensorium, even coma
- EKGs may be useful for selected patients (e.g., those with personal or family history of QTc prolongation; cardiac arrhythmia; recent myocardial infarction; uncompensated heart failure; or those taking agents that prolong QTc interval such as pimozide, thioridazine, selected antiarrhythmics, moxifloxacin, sparfloxacin, etc.)
- Patients at risk for electrolyte disturbances (e.g., patients on diuretic therapy) should have baseline and periodic serum potassium and magnesium measurements
- Patients with suspected hematologic abnormalities may require a white blood cell count before initiating treatment
- Monitor liver function tests in patients with established liver disease
- Should check blood pressure in the elderly before starting and for the first few weeks of treatment

SIDE EFFECTS

How Drug Causes Side Effects
- By blocking alpha 1 adrenergic receptors, it can cause dizziness, sedation, and hypotension
- By blocking histamine 1 receptors in the brain, it can cause sedation and weight gain
- By blocking dopamine 2 receptors in the striatum, it can cause motor side effects
- By blocking dopamine 2 receptors in the pituitary, it can cause elevations in prolactin
- Mechanism of weight gain and possible increased incidence of dyslipidemia and diabetes of atypical antipsychotics is unknown

Notable Side Effects
- Atypical antipsychotics may increase the risk for diabetes and dyslipidemia, although the specific risks associated with zotepine are unknown
- Agitation, anxiety, depression, asthenia, headache, insomnia, sedation, hypo/hyperthermia

- Constipation, dry mouth, dyspepsia, weight gain
- Tachycardia, hypotension, sweating, blurred vision
- Rare tardive dyskinesia
- Dose-related hyperprolactinemia

 ### Life Threatening or Dangerous Side Effects

- Rare neuroleptic malignant syndrome
- Rare seizures (risk increases with dose, especially over 300 mg/day)
- Blood dyscrasias
- Dose-dependent QTc prolongation
- Increased risk of death and cerebrovascular events in elderly patients with dementia-related psychosis

Weight Gain

unusual not unusual common problematic

- Many experience and/or can be significant in amount

Sedation

unusual not unusual common problematic

- Many experience and/or can be significant in amount

What To Do About Side Effects

- Wait
- Wait
- Wait
- For motor symptoms, add an anticholinergic agent
- Take more of the dose at bedtime to help reduce daytime sedation
- Weight loss, exercise programs, and medical management for high BMIs, diabetes, dyslipidemia
- Reduce the dose
- Switch to a first-line atypical antipsychotic

Best Augmenting Agents for Side Effects

- Benztropine or trihexyphenidyl for motor side effects
- Sometimes amantadine can be helpful for motor side effects
- Benzodiazepines may be helpful for akathisia
- Many side effects cannot be improved with an augmenting agent

DOSING AND USE

Usual Dosage Range

- 75–300 mg/day in 3 divided doses

Dosage Forms

- Tablet 25 mg, 50 mg, 100 mg

How to Dose

- Initial 75 mg/day in 3 doses; can increase every 4 days; maximum 300 mg/day in 3 doses

 ### Dosing Tips

- Slow initial titration can minimize hypotension
- No formal studies, but some patients may do well on twice daily dosing rather than 3 times daily dosing
- ✳ Dose-related QTc prolongation, so use with caution, especially at high doses

Overdose

- Can be fatal, especially in mixed overdoses; seizures, coma

Long-Term Use

- Can be used to delay relapse in long-term treatment of schizophrenia

Habit Forming

- No

How to Stop

- Slow down-titration (over 6 to 8 weeks), especially when simultaneously beginning a new antipsychotic while switching (i.e., cross-titration)
- Rapid discontinuation may lead to rebound psychosis and worsening of symptoms
- If antiparkinson agents are being used, they should be continued for a few weeks after zotepine is discontinued

Pharmacokinetics

- Metabolized by CYP450 3A4 and CYP450 1A2
- Active metabolite norzotepine

 ### Drug Interactions

- Combined use with phenothiazines may increase risk of seizures

- Can decrease the effects of levodopa, dopamine agonists
- Epinephrine may lower blood pressure
- May interact with hypotensive agents due to alpha 1 adrenergic blockade
- May enhance QTc prolongation of other drugs capable of prolonging QTc interval
- Plasma concentrations increased by diazepam, fluoxetine
- Zotepine may increase plasma levels of phenytoin
- May increase risk of bleeding if used with anticoagulants
- Theoretically, dose may need to be raised if given in conjunction with CYP450 1A2 inducers (e.g., cigarette smoke)
- Theoretically, dose may need to be lowered if given in conjunction with CYP450 1A2 inhibitors (e.g., fluvoxamine) in order to prevent dangers of dose-dependent QTc prolongation
- Theoretically, dose may need to be lowered if given in conjunction with CYP450 3A4 inhibitors (e.g., fluvoxamine, nefazodone, fluoxetine) in order to prevent dangers of dose-dependent QTc prolongation

⚠ Other Warnings/ Precautions

- Not recommended for use with sibutramine
- Use cautiously in patients with alcohol withdrawal or convulsive disorders because of possible lowering of seizure threshold
- If signs of neuroleptic malignant syndrome develop, treatment should be immediately discontinued
- Because zotepine may dose-dependently prolong QTc interval, use with caution in patients who have bradycardia or who are taking drugs that can induce bradycardia (e.g., beta blockers, calcium channel blockers, clonidine, digitalis)
- Because zotepine may dose-dependently prolong QTc interval, use with caution in patients who have hypokalemia and or hypomagnesemia or who are taking drugs than can induce hypokalemia and/or magnesemia (e.g., diuretics, stimulant laxatives, intravenous amphotericin B, glucocorticoids, tetracosactide)
- Because zotepine dose-dependently prolongs QTc interval, use with caution in patients taking any agent capable of

increasing zotepine plasma levels (e.g., diazepam, CYP450 1A2 inhibitors and CYP450 3A4 inhibitors)

Do Not Use

- If patient has epilepsy or family history of epilepsy
- If patient has gout or history of nephrolithiasis
- If patient is taking other CNS depressants
- If patient is taking high doses of other antipsychotics
- If patient is taking agents capable of significantly prolonging QTc interval (e.g., pimozide; thioridazine; selected antiarrhythmics such as quinidine, disopyramide, amiodarone, and sotalol; selected antibiotics such as moxifloxacin and sparfloxacin)
- If there is a history of QTc prolongation or cardiac arrhythmia, recent acute myocardial infarction, uncompensated heart failure
- If patient is pregnant or breast feeding
- If there is a proven allergy to zotepine

SPECIAL POPULATIONS

Renal Impairment

- Recommended starting dose 25 mg twice a day; recommended maximum dose generally 75 mg twice a day

Hepatic Impairment

- Recommended starting dose 25 mg twice a day; recommended maximum dose generally 75 mg twice a day
- May require weekly monitoring of liver function during the first few months of treatment

Cardiac Impairment

- Drug should be used with caution
- Zotepine produces a dose-dependent prolongation of QTc interval, which may be enhanced by the existence of bradycardia, hypokalemia, congenital or acquired long QTc interval, which should be evaluated prior to administering zotepine
- Use with caution if treating concomitantly with a medication likely to produce prolonged bradycardia, hypokalemia, slowing of intracardiac conduction, or prolongation of the QTc interval

- Avoid zotepine in patients with a known history of QTc prolongation, recent acute myocardial infraction, and uncompensated heart failure

Elderly

- Recommended starting dose 25 mg twice a day; recommended maximum dose generally 75 mg twice a day
- Although atypical antipsychotics are commonly used for behavioral disturbances in dementia, no agent has been approved for treatment of elderly patients with dementia-related psychosis
- Elderly patients with dementia-related psychosis treated with atypical antipsychotics are at an increased risk of death compared to placebo, and also have an increased risk of cerebrovascular events

 Children and Adolescents

- Not recommended under age 18

 Pregnancy

- Insufficient data in humans to determine risk
- Zotepine is not recommended during pregnancy

Breast Feeding

- Zotepine is not recommended during breast feeding
- Immediate postpartum period is a high-risk time for relapse of psychosis, so may consider treatment with another antipsychotic

THE ART OF PSYCHOPHARMACOLOGY

Potential Advantages

- Norepinephrine reuptake blocking actions have theoretical benefits for cognition (attention) and for depression

Potential Disadvantages

- Patients not compliant with 3 times daily dosing
- Patients requiring rapid onset of antipsychotic action
- Patients with uncontrolled seizures

Primary Target Symptoms

- Positive symptoms of psychosis
- Negative symptoms of psychosis
- Cognitive functioning
- Depressive symptoms

 Pearls

* Zotepine inhibits norepinephrine reuptake, which may have implications for treatment of depression, as well as for cognitive symptoms of schizophrenia
- Risks of diabetes and dyslipidemia not well-studied for zotepine, but known significant weight gain suggests the need for careful monitoring during zotepine treatment
- Not as well investigated in bipolar disorder, but its mechanism of action suggests efficacy in acute bipolar mania

 Suggested Reading

Ackenheil M. [The biochemical effect profile of zotepine in comparison with other neuroleptics]. Fortschr Neurol Psychiatr 1991; 59 Suppl 1: 2–9.

Fenton M, Morris S, De-Silva P, Bagnall A, Cooper SJ, Gammelin G, Leitner M. Zotepine for schizophrenia. Cochrane Database Syst Rev 2000; (2): CD001948.

Stanniland C, Taylor D. Tolerability of atypical antipsychotics. Drug Saf 2000; 22 (3): 195–214.

Index by Drug Name

Index by Use

Bold for FDA approved

Aggression
  clozapine, *19*

Anxiety
  cyamemazine, *25*
  gabapentin (adjunct), *31*
  pregabalin, *71*

Behavioral problems
  aripiprazole, *7*
  olanzapine, *55*
  quetiapine, *75*
  risperidone, *81*
  ziprasidone, *101*

Bipolar depression
  aripiprazole, *7*
  carbamazepine, *13*
  lamotrigine, *37*
  lithium, *49*
  olanzapine, *55*
  olanzapine-fluoxetine combination, *55*
  quetiapine, *75*
  risperidone, *81*
  valproate (divalproex), *95*
  ziprasidone, *101*

Bipolar disorder
  aripiprazole, *7*
  carbamazepine, *13*
  cyamemazine, *25*
  gabapentin (adjunct), *31*
  lamotrigine, *37*
  levetiracetam, *45*
  lithium, *49*
  olanzapine, *55*
  olanzapine-fluoxetine combination, *55*
  oxcarbazepine, *61*
  quetiapine, *75*
  risperidone, *81*
  topiramate (adjunct), *89*
  valproate (divalproex), *95*
  ziprasidone, *101*
  zonisamide, *107*
  zotepine, *111*

Bipolar maintenance
  aripiprazole, *7*
  carbamazepine, *13*
  lamotrigine, *37*
  lithium, *49*
  olanzapine, *55*

olanzapine-fluoxetine combination, *55*
quetiapine, *75*
risperidone, *81*
valproate (divalproex), *95*
ziprasidone, *101*

Bulimia nervosa/binge eating
  topiramate, *89*
  zonisamide, *107*

Depression
  amisulpride, *1*
  cyamemazine, *25*
  lithium (adjunct), *49*
  olanzapine, *55*

Fibromyalgia
  pregabalin, *71*

Generalized anxiety disorder
  pregabalin, *71*

Glossopharyngeal neuralgia
  carbamazepine, *13*

Mania
  aripiprazole, *7*
  carbamazepine, *13*
  lamotrigine, *37*
  levetiracetam, *45*
  lithium, *49*
  olanzapine, *55*
  quetiapine, *75*
  risperidone, *81*
  valproate (divalproex), *95*
  ziprasidone, *101*
  zotepine, *111*

Migraine
  topiramate, *89*
  valproate (divalproex), *95*

Neuropathic pain/chronic pain
  carbamazepine, *13*
  gabapentin, *31*
  lamotrigine, *37*
  levetiracetam, *45*
  pregabalin, *71*
  topiramate, *89*
  valproate (divalproex), *95*
  zonisamide, *107*

Abbreviations

5HT	serotonin
ACH	acetylcholine
ACHE	acetylcholinesterase
ADHD	attention deficit hyperactivity disorder
ALT	alanine aminotransferase
ALPT	total serum alkaline phosphatase
AST	aspartate aminotransferase
BID	twice a day
BMI	body mass index
BuChE	butyrylcholinesterase
CMI	clomipramine
CNS	central nervous system
CYP450	cytochrome P450
De-CMI	desmethyl-clomipramine
DA	dopamine
dl	deciliter
DLB	dementia with Lewy bodies
DPNP	diabetic peripheral neuropathic pain
ECG	electrocardiogram
EEG	electroencephalogram
EKG	electrocardiogram
EPS	extrapyramidal side effects
ERT	estrogen replacement therapy
FDA	Food and Drug Administration
FSH	follicle-stimulating hormone
GAD	generalized anxiety disorder
GI	gastrointestinal
HDL	high-density lipoprotein
HMG CoA	beta-hydroxy-beta-methylglutaryl Coenzyme A
HRT	hormone replacement therapy
IM	intramuscular
IV	intravenous
LDL	low-density lipoprotein
LH	luteinizing hormone
Lb	pound
MAO	monoamine oxidase
MAOI	monoamine oxidase inhibitor
mCPP	meta-chloro-phenyl-piperazine
mg	milligram
mL	milliliter
mm Hg	millimeters of mercury

MDD	major depressive disorder
NE	norepinephrine
NMDA	N-methyl-d-aspartate
OCD	obsessive-compulsive disorder
ODV	O-desmethylvenlafaxine
PET	positron emission tomography
PK	pharmacokinetic
PMDD	premenstrual dysphoric disorder
PMS	premenstrual syndrome
PTSD	posttraumatic stress disorder
QD	once a day
QHS	once a day at bedtime
QID	four times a day
RIMA	reversible inhibitor of monoamine oxidase A
SNRI	dual serotonin and norepinephrine reuptake inhibitor
SSRI	selective serotonin reuptake inhibitor
TCA	tricyclic antidepressant
TID	three times a day
TSH	thyroid stimulating hormone

FDA Use-In-Pregnancy Ratings

Category A: Controlled studies show no risk: adequate, well-controlled studies in pregnant women have failed to demonstrate risk to the fetus

Category B: No evidence of risk in humans: either animal findings show risk, but human findings do not; or, if no adequate human studies have been performed, animal findings are negative

Category C: Risk cannot be ruled out: human studies are lacking, and animal studies are either positive for fetal risk or lacking as well. However, potential benefits may outweigh risks

Category D: Positive evidence of risk: investigational or postmarketing data show risk to the fetus. Nevertheless, potential benefits may outweigh risks

Category X: Contraindicated in pregnancy: studies in animals or humans, or investigational or postmarketing reports, have shown fetal risk that clearly outweighs any possible benefit to the patient